An Introduction to the U.S. Health Care System

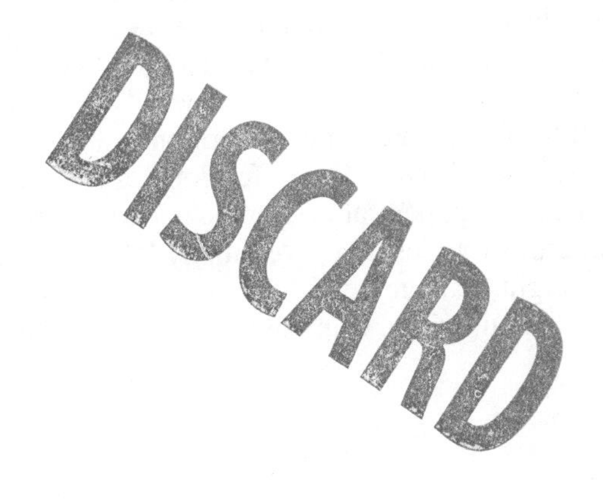

Steven Jonas, MD, MPH, is Professor of Preventive Medicine, School of Medicine, State University of New York at Stony Brook, where he has been a faculty member since 1971. Born and raised in New York City, he received his B.A. from Columbia College in 1958, his M.D. from the Harvard Medical School in 1962, his M.P.H. from the Yale School of Medicine in 1967, and his M.S. in Health Management from New York University in 1997.

He is a Fellow of the American College of Preventive Medicine, the American Public Health Association, and the New York Academy of Medicine. He is Editor of the Springer *Series on Medical Education*, an Associate Editor of *Preventive Medicine*, and a member of the Editorial Board of the *American Journal of Preventive Medicine*. He is a Past President of the Association of Teachers of Preventive Medicine and a past member of the New York State Board for Medicine.Dr. Jonas is Founding Editor of *Jonas-Kovner: Health Care Delivery in the United States* (published by Springer), was Editor and coauthor of its first three editions, and is Coeditor of the Sixth Edition (forthcoming in 1998). He has authored seven books of his own, including *Quality Control of Ambulatory Care* (published by Springer, 1977), *Medical Mystery: The Training of Doctors in the United States* (New York: W. W. Norton, 1978), and *The Essential Triathlete* (New York: Lyons and Burford, 1996). He is author or coauthor of seven books on exercise and weight management.

On health policy, preventive medicine, and drug abuse policy, Dr. Jonas has published over 100 professional articles and book reviews and delivered over 75 papers at conferences and seminars. He has also published numerous articles and given many talks on sports, exercise promotion, and weight management. He was a designated speaker on behalf of the National Health Care Campaign for the Clinton Health Plan in 1994.

An Introduction to the U.S. Health Care System

Fourth Edition

Steven Jonas

MD, MPH, FACPM

1st and 2nd Editions by ***Milton Roemer****, MD, MPH*

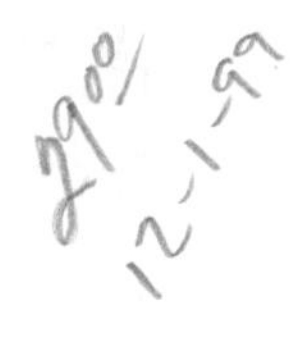

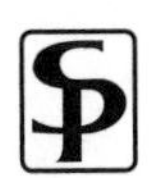 **Springer Publishing Company**

Springer Publishing Company, Inc.
536 Broadway
New York, NY 10012-3955

Cover design by Margaret Dunin
Acquisitions Editor: Matt Fenton
Production Editor: Kathleen Kelly

98 99 00 01 02/5 4 3

Library of Congress Cataloging-in-Publication Data

Jonas, Steven.
An introduction to the U.S. health care system / Steven Jonas.
p. cm.
Includes bibliographical references and index.
ISBN 0-8261-3985-X
1. Medical care—United States. I. Title.
RA395.A3J654 1997
362.1'0973—dc21 97-24632
CIP

Printed in the United States of America

For my mother,
Mrs. Florence Kyzor Jonas,
born February 8, 1908

Contents

Foreword to the Fourth Edition **ix**
Preface to the Fourth Edition **xi**
Abbreviations **xii**

Chapter 1 An Overview of the U.S. Health Care System 1
Chapter 2 Personnel 25
Chapter 3 Institutions: Hospitals 45
Chapter 4 Institutions: Primary and Ambulatory Care 63
Chapter 5 Financing 84
Chapter 6 Government 103
Chapter 7 Principles of Health Planning 123
Chapter 8 From Group Medical Practice to Managed Care 144
Chapter 9 National Health Insurance and National Health Reform 165
Appendix I 189
Appendix II 191
Index *197*

Foreword

The United States health care system is in the midst of significant change due to a confluence of public sector and private sector forces. Ironically, the failed Clinton Health Reform legislation of 1994 may have resulted in more change than would have occurred with its passage. Certainly, there has been greater diversity of change than what would have occurred otherwise. For those trying to learn about the health care system in the United States, there is a great need to understand the complex forces, issues, and values involved. It is also important to be able to place the issues in historical context, as the "issues of the moment" do not arise totally independent from what has gone before. An introductory text to the field needs to be reasonably comprehensive, integrative, provide an appropriate historical context, focus on the most important issues, provide a way of analyzing the issues, and, if possible, be interesting. *An Introduction to the U. S. Health Care System, 4th Edition,* by Steve Jonas succeeds on all of these criteria.

Perhaps the most fundamental insight into how we do things in the United States is to understand our "incremental" approach. We tend to creep up on things doing a little bit here and a little bit there and wait to see what happens. Above all, we tend to protect our long-cherished values of autonomy, choice, and individualism, even if, at times, they make it difficult to develop a sense of community, a shared common vision for our health care system, or a sense of collective social justice. One senses from reading this text a certain impatience on the part of the author perhaps stemming from the fact that many seemingly workable solutions to our health care problems were identified long ago in the Report of the Committee on the Costs of Medical Care in 1932. This "impatience" provides the book with a bit of an "edge" and, in my view, increases its interest for the reader.

This book has many strengths. Among its most prominent is its treatment of the historical forces leading up to the contemporary health policy issues. These issues are framed with just the right amount of historical context provided, without getting carried away in details of little interest or use. Chapter 1 also provides relevant comparisons to other countries and thus avoids the parochialism often found with introductory texts on the U.S. health care system. Chapter 5 offers a useful overview of financing options and issues. Dr. Jonas reminds us that the pluralistic approaches and options reflect our underlying values of autonomy and choice, even if they create inefficiencies and, at times, perverse incentives. We get what we want. Chapter 6 provides an excellent description and analysis of the role of government agencies at all levels including the Centers for Disease Control, the Office of Disease Prevention and Health Promotion, other branches of the service, the Veterans Administration, the Department of Defense, and the responsibilities of state agencies. Chapter 7 reminds readers that planning cannot be effective without a direct linkage to the flow of funds—a message that is reiterated in Chapter 9 dealing with National Health Insurance and health reform. The book also contains a new chapter on managed care (Chapter 10) highlighting some of the issues posed by the growing for-profit role in health care delivery. A special feature is a Guide to Sources of Data provided in Appendix II.

This book is well-suited to its primary audiences—undergraduate students, medical and health professions students, and those with a general interest in learning more about the U.S. health care system. It succeeds in challenging readers to form their own conclusions regarding the issues and information presented, but one suspects that Dr. Jonas would like his readers to go one step beyond forming their own conclusions and that is to take *action*! The current cohort of health professional students, future policy makers, and would-be executives will have unparalleled opportunities to put their own stamp on the evolving U.S. health care system providing the ''grist'' for future editions of this book.

STEPHEN M. SHORTELL, PH.D.
A.C. Buehler Distinguished Professor of Health Services Management and
Professor of Organization Behavior
J.L. Kellogg Graduate School of Management and
Institute for Health Services Research and Policy Studies
Northwestern University, Evanston, Illinois

Preface

This is the fourth edition of *An Introduction to the U.S. Health Care System*. In keeping with Dr. Milton Roemer's original intention for the first edition, the book describes the U.S. health care delivery system in broad outline. It was my privilege, and indeed an honor, with the third edition to have succeeded Dr. Roemer as the principal author of this book.

In 1966, then a student at the Yale School of Public Health, I went to my first American Public Health Association Annual Meeting. My mentor, the late Dr. E. Richard Weinerman, introduced me to all the luminaries of the field that was then called ''Medical Care.'' None shone more brightly than Dr. Roemer. When we began our work together on the third edition of this book, I felt like the kid who idolized the super-star baseball player and then grew up to play on the same team with him.

The third edition of *An Introduction* was a substantial revision of Dr. Roemer's previous edition, but did draw significantly on that work. The bulk of the writing in this Fourth Edition is my own. Any of Dr. Roemer's text that still remains in this edition is used with the kind permission of Dr. Roemer, and with my thanks to him.

This book focuses on principles, basic structures, and important unsolved problems. It is not concerned with the specifics of current legislative proposals and programs and how they are or are not being implemented. It takes a mainly qualitative, rather than quantitative, approach. Statistics and citations are used sparingly, and, while referenced, it does not have a profusion of citations. For a more comprehensive approach, more quantitative information, and many more references, readers are directed to *Health Care Delivery in the United States*.*

**Health Care Delivery in the United States* provides in-depth description and analysis of the subject, in contrast with the introductory approach that this book takes. Earlier versions of certain portions of the text written by me for this book appeared in parts that I wrote of the 2nd, 3rd, and to a very limited extent the 4th, editions of Health Care Delivery in the United States. That text is used with the permission of the publisher and copyright holder, the Springer Publishing Co. I edited the 2nd and 3rd editions of HCDUS, published in 1981 and 1986, respectively. The 4th and 5th editions were edited by my friend and colleague Anthony Kovner, Ph.D., and published in 1990 and 1995. The 6th edition, coedited by Dr. Kovner and myself, is scheduled for publication in 1998.

As were the first three editions, this book is primarily intended for use in undergraduate courses on the U.S. health care delivery system, in graduate survey courses, for teaching the subject to medical students (who usually do not cover it in any depth, if they cover it at all), and for the practicing health professional who simply wants an overview of the system.

Although *An Introduction* is not a policy book, both Dr. Roemer and I have written a great deal on policy. Thus, this book has a political and philosophical point of view. It always attempts to be objective, but it is not neutral. The material is presented from the position that the principal purpose of the U.S. health care delivery system is to meet and serve the health care needs of the American people.

At various points in the book, especially in Chapters 8 and 9, proposals for U.S. health care delivery system policy and program changes are described. Some proposals are recommended. I hope that, after assimilating the factual material presented, you will be able to come to your own conclusions about what change is needed, if any. I am certain that, if nothing else, you will agree with the majority of the American people that both the structure and the functions of the system must be reformed.

As in previous editions, the book's structure remains rather straightforward. Chapter 1 provides an overview of the system. Chapter 2 presents the people who provide the care. Chapters 3 and 4 cover the system's primary inpatient and outpatient institutions and institutional forms. Financing is reviewed in Chapter 5. Chapter 6 covers governmental roles and functions, and Chapter 7, the principles of health planning. New to the book is Chapter 8, entirely devoted to the subject of managed care. The history of and prospects for national health insurance in the United States are discussed in Chapter 9.

I am pleased to acknowledge the support of my Department Chairman, Dr. M. Cristina Leske, for this project. Many thanks to my friends at the photocopying center, Health Sciences Center, SUNY at Stony Brook. At Springer, I thank Pam Lankas, Louise Farkas, Matt Fenton and Bill Tucker, Rose Pintaudi, Ed Hanus, and last, but never least, the woman without whom none of this work would ever have seen the light of day, Dr. Ursula Springer, President of the Springer Publishing Company.

Abbreviations

AALL	—	American Association for Labor Legislation
AAMC	—	Association of American Medical Colleges
AHA	—	American Hospital Association
AIDS	—	Acquired Immuno-Deficiency Syndrome
ALOS	—	Average Length of Stay
AMA	—	American Medical Association
ANA	—	American Nurses' Association
ASTHO	—	Association of State and Territorial Health Officials
CAT	—	Computerized Axial Tomography
CCMC	—	Committee on the Costs of Medical Care
CDCP	—	Centers for Disease Control and Prevention
CHC	—	Community Health Center
CHP	—	Comprehensive Health Planning or Clinton Health Plan (check context)
CHSS	—	Cooperative Health Statistics System
CME	—	Continuing Medical Education
CPO	—	Combined Provider Organization
DHEW	—	Department of Health, Education and Welfare
DHHS	—	Department of Health and Human Services
D.O.	—	Doctor of Osteopathy
DOD	—	Department of Defense
DRG	—	Diagnosis Related Group
DVA	—	Department of Veterans Affairs
EAP	—	Employee Assistance Program
ED	—	Emergency Department
EMS	—	Emergency Medical Service (or System)
EMT	—	Emergency Medical Technician
EPA	—	Environmental Protection Agency
EPO	—	Exclusive Provider Organization
FDA	—	Food and Drug Administration
GAO	—	General Accounting Office
GDP	—	Gross Domestic Product

GMENAC — Graduate Medical Education National Advisory Committee
GNP — Gross National Product
GPEP — General Professional Education of the Physician Panel
HANES — Health and Nutrition Examination Survey
HCDS — Health Care Delivery System
HCFA — Health Care Financing Administration
HHS — Health and Human Services
HI — Hospital Insurance
HIP — Health Insurance Plan
HIV — Human Immunodeficiency Virus
HMO — Health Maintenance Organization
HRA — Health Resources Administration; Health Risk Appraisal (check context)
HRSA — Health Resources and Services Administration
HSA — Health Systems Agency
IDS — Integrated Delivery System
IPA — Individual or Independent Practice Association
IPO — Independent Practice Organization
JCAH — Joint Commission on Accreditation of Hospitals
LCME — Liaison Committee on Medical Education
LHD — Local Health Department
LPN — Licensed Practical Nurse
M.C. — Managed Care
MCH — Maternal and Child Health
MCO — Managed Care Organization
MHS — Marine Hospital Service
MMWR — *Morbidity and Mortality Weekly Report*
MRI — Magnetic Resonance Imaging
MVSR — *Monthly Vital Statistics Report*
NCHS — National Center for Health Statistics
NE — Nurse Extender
NHC — Neighborhood Health Center
NHI — National Health Insurance
NHS — National Health Survey or Service (check the context)
NIH — National Institutes of Health
NIMH — National Institute of Mental Health
NIOSH — National Institute of Occupational Safety and Health
NLN — National League for Nursing
NP — Nurse Practitioner
ODPHP — Office of Disease Prevention and Health Promotion
OEO — Office of Economic Opportunity

OMB	—	Office of Management and Budget
OPD	—	Out-Patient Department
OSHA	—	Occupational Safety and Health Administration
PA	—	Physicians' Assistant (or Associate)
PHCS	—	Personal Health Care System
PHO	—	Physician Hospital Organization
PHS	—	Public Health Service
POS	—	Point of Service
PPGP	—	Prepaid Group Practice
PPO	—	Preferred Provider Organization
RBRVS	—	Resource Based Relative Value System
RCT	—	Registered Care Technician
RMP	—	Regional Medical Programs
RN	—	Registered Nurse
SAMSHA	—	Substance Abuse and Mental Health Services Administration
SHA	—	State Health Agency
SMI	—	Supplementary Medical Insurance
STD	—	Sexually Transmitted Disease
TB	—	Tuberculosis
UR	—	Ut ilization Review
USDA	—	United States Department of Agriculture
USDHEW	—	United States Department of Health, Education and Welfare
USDHHS	—	United States Department of Health and Human Services
USGPO	—	United States Government Printing Office
USPHS	—	United States Public Health Service
VA	—	Veterans Administration
WHO	—	World Health Organization
WIC	—	Women and Infants Care

Chapter 1

An Overview of the U.S. Health Care System

MAJOR DEFINING CHARACTERISTICS

The International Context

A colleague once said of health maintenance organizations (HMOs) (Kodner, 1996): ''When you've seen one HMO, you've seen one HMO.'' The same could be said of the health care systems of the nations of the world. No two are exactly the same. Yet those of most of the major industrialized countries do share common features (Roemer, 1991, 1993), except for the health care system of the United States of America. Even among the industrialized nations its system is unique. It is thus a truism that: ''When you have seen the U.S. health care system, you've seen the U.S. health care system.''

As we begin to examine this system it is helpful to place some of its features in the context of the health care systems of the other major industrialized countries. Indeed there are several major characteristics of the system of health care in the United States that distinguish it not only from that of the other industrialized countries but from that of all of the world's 160 or so other nations.

First, the United States spends a higher proportion of its gross domestic product on health services than does any other country in the world: 13.7% in 1994 (Levit, 1996). Second, alone among the world's industrialized countries, the United States does not have a comprehensive system for paying for health services for all or most of the residents of the country (national health insurance), let alone a comprehensive national health system.

Third, although private fee-for-service medical practice of a sort that produced, among other things, high incomes for many physicians has existed in the United States for decades (a feature shared to a greater or lesser extent with a number of countries that do have some form of national health *insurance*), recently the U.S. health care system has become a major venue for the generation of corporate profits from the direct provision of health care services. This too is a unique feature of the U.S. health care system.

Finally, the distribution of and access to health services for the American people is significantly uneven (Wennberg et al., 1996). For many people who live in the right geographic location, have the right health-care-cost-coverage package, and have a disease or condition on which American medicine has chosen to focus, American medicine is, as it is said, "The best in the world." But for the person who lives in the wrong place (Wennberg et al., 1996), with no health care cost coverage (Donelan et al., 1996), who is, for example, someone other than a young white male (Geiger, 1996), and worse yet has a disease or condition in which American medicine has limited interest, that may well not be true. Such a person may be in serious trouble in terms of both his or her health care and his or her health.

The Role of the Market

Economic markets exist for the purpose of allocating scarce resources to pay for the provision of goods and services. A major defining characteristic of the U.S. health care system is the centrality of its operations in the form of what is generally called the "free market" (Ginzberg, 1996). A primary defining characteristic of the free market is that it is at its base profit-driven (Lehman, 1996). That is, although a variety of social goods and needs can be served by the operation of a free market, its primary goal is the production of private profit from the very process of allocating scarce resources to pay for the provision of goods and services (Sherill, 1995).

In contrast to the free market stands what might be called the "social/community market." A primary defining characteristic of this market is that it is at its base use-driven. That is, although private profit for some may result from the operation of a social/community market, its primary goal is to provide for the equitable, effective, and efficient use of the scarce resources that are being allocated to pay for goods and services. Thus although the free market is driven in the first instance by private profit (or at a less complex level simple private income accumulation), the social/community market is driven in the first instance by broader individual, community, and social values.

In the United States over the course of the 20th century, a good deal of political and financial capital has been spent maintaining the primacy of place of the free market in the health care delivery system. This has resulted in a largely successful ongoing campaign to minimize "government interference in the practice of medicine" and a completely successful ongoing campaign to "prevent a government takeover" of the U.S. health care system.

As of the writing of this book, the most recent iteration of the latter was the 1994 defeat in Congress of the Clinton Health Plan (see chapter 9) by its political opponents and those insurance, hospital, pharmaceutical, and medical interests opposed to the creation of a single national (although ironically not government-run [DPC, 1993]) health system. Those interests very effectively provided financial, logistical, and intellectual support to the Plan's political opponents. The "free market" for the health care system was preserved once again.

Changes in the Physician-Patient Relationship

Traditionally, in accordance with its "free market" ethic, American medical practice has been organized primarily on the private entrepreneurial model (see chapter 2). With the advent of managed care (see chapter 8) that pattern is changing (Kassirer, 1995). Traditionally, whether or not the service was paid for by the patient or a third party other than the patient or physician, medical care in the United States has been provided primarily on the basis of a private, direct (usually unwritten) contract between physician and patient. In the present era, more and more it is a corporation, a managed care organization (MCO), most of which are of the for-profit type (Fubini, 1996), which contracts with patients, either directly or through their employers, to provide their medical care.

Traditionally, American physicians have controlled the bulk of the decision-making process concerning the allocation and use of health care system resources, whether through visits to the physicians themselves, diagnostic tests, hospital admissions, surgical interventions, use of pharmaceuticals, or others. One of the major factors leading to the ever-rising costs of U.S. health care (Levit, 1996, Fig. 1) has been this characteristic of independent physician decision making in resource allocation.

As MCOs increasingly become the primary contractor with patients for the provision of medical care, they are taking control of the decision-making authority from the physicians over how health care system resources are utilized and spent. This has led to a certain degree of cost containment, as utilization of certain resources has declined (KPMG, 1996). But it has also led to a rising level of unhappiness and dissatisfaction, for somewhat different reasons, among both doctors and patients (*Consumer Reports*, 1996). These are some of the themes to which we shall return at various points in this book. But now let us consider an overview of the U.S. health care system, beginning with some of the characteristics of the population that it serves.

THE HEALTH STATUS OF THE U.S. POPULATION

In 1995 the United States population was about 263 million (*Stat*, 1996, Table 2).[1] Many ethnic and national groups are represented and a broad range of social classes with large income differentials (that are becoming wider over time [Thurow, 1995]) exist. There are also significant differences in health status between population subgroups (Adler et al., 1995; Pappas et al., 1993). Proportionately, there are more non-White persons in the lower social class and income groups than in the general population. Unemployment or the threat of it, substandard housing, and dysnutrition are major socioeconomic problems in rural as well as urban areas.

The projected 1993 life expectancy at birth for U.S. residents was 75.5 years (*Stat*, 1996, Table 119). For men it was 72.3 years, whereas for women it was 78.8 years. In 1995, close to 13% of the population consisted of persons 65 and over (*Stat*, 1996, Table 14). There was a marked difference in life expectancy at birth by race (projected, 1995): 77.0 for Whites, 72.5 for Blacks (*Stat*, 1996, Table 118). The Black–White difference in life expectancy is thought in part to reflect differences in the standard of living, as well as access to health services (Schwartz et al., 1990).

In 1995 (projected) the U.S. infant mortality rate was 6.7 per 1,000 live births (*Stat*, 1996, Table 1327). Although this is low, of course, it is slightly higher than that of some 11 other countries, mainly in Western Europe, but including Australia, Canada, and Japan (*Stat*, 1996, Table 1327). It is perhaps significant that in 1994 other than Denmark, Japan,

---

[1]Unless otherwise referenced, the data presented in the balance of this chapter come from the *Statistical Abstract of the United States*, 116th ed., (Washington, DC: U.S. Bureau of the Census, 1996, cited in the text as *Stat*), and *Health United States*, 1995, (Hyattsville, MD: U.S. Department of Health and Human Services [USDHHS], Pub. No. [PHS] 96-1232, May, 1996, cited in the text as *Health*). The year given in the text for each datum is the most recent one for which that information is available.

and Switzerland, these countries had a lower *per capita* gross national product than does the U.S. (*Stat*, 1996, Table 1334). Nevertheless, they all have systems of national health care that make services accessible to virtually everyone at little or no cost at the time of service.

The White/Black difference in infant mortality rate in the U.S. is striking. In 1994 it was 6.6 for Whites, 15.8 for Blacks (Singh et al., 1996, p. 10). The Black infant mortality rate has been at least double that for Whites since 1915 when the rate was first recorded and it was 99.9 overall (Grove & Hetzel, 1968). In 1994 the crude death rate was 8.8 per 1,000 population, 9.2 for males, 8.4 for females (Singh et al., 1996, Table 1). Again, there was a major differential by ethnic group. The *crude* death rate was higher for Whites, 9.1, than it was for Blacks, 8.6. But the *age-adjusted* death rates (''age-adjustment'' statistically accounts for the fact that life expectancy for Blacks is shorter than for Whites) were 4.8 for Whites, 7.7 for Blacks.

As of 1994 the 15 leading causes of death characterized by diagnosed disease or condition in the general population were heart disease, cancer, stroke, chronic obstructive lung disease, personal injury (''accidents''), pneumonia, diabetes mellitus, human immunodeficiency virus (HIV) infection, suicide, chronic liver disease and cirrhosis, homicide and ''legal intervention'' (execution), kidney disease, blood infection, Alzheimer's disease, and atherosclerosis (Singh et al., 1996, Table B).

Looking at the ''cause of death'' in a rather different way, that is, by major contributing cause of the disease(s) to which the death was attributed rather than by the disease(s) themselves, as of 1990 the leading factors were (McGinnis & Foege, 1993): tobacco use, dietary patterns, sedentary lifestyle, alcohol consumption, microbial agents, toxic agents, firearms, sexual behavior, motor vehicles, and use of the illicit drugs.

As of 1995 the major causes of morbidity (sickness) were upper respiratory infections, influenza, injuries, other infective and parasitic diseases, chronic sinusitis, arthritis, hypertension, heart conditions, orthopedic impairments (including low back pain), and asthma and hay fever (Adams & Marano, 1995, Tables 2, 57).

Considering some of the social factors related to ill health, there is no consistent association between family income and the number of acute conditions per 100 persons per year (Adams & Marano, 1995, Table 4). There is an inverse correlation between family income and the number of days of restricted activity associated with acute conditions (Adams & Marano, 1995, Table 19), however. It is interesting to note that Blacks report both fewer acute conditions and fewer days of restricted activity related to them than do Whites (Adams & Marano, 1995, Tables 3, 18).

THE ELEMENTS OF THE SYSTEM

Introduction

Any health care delivery system has five major components: the health care institutions, the personnel who work in them, the firms producing "health commodities" such as pharmaceutical drugs and hospital equipment, the research and educational institutions that produce biomedical knowledge and health personnel, and the financing mechanism. In addition, in the other developed and numerous less developed countries an organizational structure stands at the system's center, like the trunk of a tree. There are other loci of power and control, to be sure. But the organizational structure is the central one. It enables the system's components to interact and function to produce health services for the people. In the U.S. as already noted there is no central trunk, but multiple ones. For the U.S., think Banyan tree, not oak.

In this regard, as with the other characteristics noted at the beginning of this chapter, among the industrialized countries of the world, the U.S. system is once again unique. As one would expect, there is no national Ministry of Health playing a central role in the operation and/or financing of health services. In the other industrialized countries, even if the Ministry does not operate the health care system directly, at the least it creates and supervises the structure within which it functions. The Ministry of Health or its equivalent customarily runs the national system for paying for health care.

In the United States there is, of course, a health care *system*—just not a national one with a recognizable structure. Care is provided and it is paid for. There is a (highly complex and confusing, not in any way completely understood) management structure. Top quality health sciences research and education are carried out. There are certainly loci of power and control. But they are sometimes difficult to recognize and to describe. Nevertheless, it can be safely said that it is amazing, as noted above, how much money and time the principal loci of power and control have spent to make sure that the U.S. does not have a single national structure for paying for, much less operating its health care system.

Health Services Components

In this section we briefly consider each of the five major components of the health care delivery system: personnel, institutions, commodities, knowledge and personnel production, and financing. (The principal ones are further treated in separate chapters.)

Health Personnel

In 1994, about 10.6 million people worked in the health care delivery system (*Health*, 1996, Table 96). The largest groups are the nurses, clerical staff, hospital manual workers, physicians, pharmacists, dentists, and technicians (*Health*, 1996, Table 101). The physicians, of whom there were about 630,000 active in 1993, traditionally have been the most powerful, dominant group. In the mid-1990s, as noted, a major change of the locus of control was taking place, as it moved to the managed care companies. (Health manpower is covered in chapter 2.)

Health Care Institutions

Of the institutions housing and caring for patients in bed, acute-care hospitals are the most numerous. In 1993, there were about 5,600 of them, with about 990,000 beds (*Health*, 1996, Table 107). Hospitals are categorized in a variety of ways: by ownership, size, function, and average length of patient stay.

There are three principal types of ownership: government (federal, state, and local); private, not for profit (voluntary); and private, for profit (proprietary). There are four functional categories: general, mental, rehabilitation and chronic disease, and "other special" (AHA, 1995, p. A5). The American Hospital Association also defines the "community hospital," as a nonfederal, short-term general or other special hospital. This is the predominant type of hospital in the United States. (Hospitals are covered in chapter 3. Nursing homes and other nonmental-condition long-term care institutions, of which there were about 15,000 in 1991 [*Health*, 1996, Table 113], plus other long-term care services, are briefly described in chapter 3.)

Various types of institutions provide other types of health care services. The most frequently used type of care is described as "ambulatory." Ambulatory care is that provided to patients other than those in institutional beds. About 60% of ambulatory care is delivered in private doctors' offices; other sites include hospital ambulatory services (about 13%), by telephone (about 14%), the home (about 1.5%), and "other" (group practices, health maintenance organizations, neighborhood health centers, and local health department health centers), about 13% (*Health*, 1996, Table 64). (For more detail on ambulatory services, see chapter 4.)

Health Commodities

A wide variety of commodities is used in the health care delivery system. Many kinds of equipment and supplies for the diagnosis and treatment of disease are produced by the hospital and medical supply manufacturers. These items range from gauze pads, hospital furniture, sterile needles, laboratory chemicals, and anesthetic gases, to diagnostic imaging and laboratory equipment, surgical instruments, orthopedic appliances, eyeglasses, hearing aids, and dental prostheses. The other major category of health commodity is pharmaceutical drugs. These elements, as important as they are, are not covered in any detail in this book.

The Reproduction of Health Personnel and Knowledge

The scientific basis of every health care system is the fund of knowledge about health and disease, and the understanding of how to apply that knowledge to prevention and treatment through various technologies. A vast store of knowledge, of course, has been gathered from the observations and experience of past centuries. In our era both the scientific knowledge base and our understanding of the best means for applying it to health maintenance and disease treatment are expanding at an ever-increasing rate. This is the primary function of the biomedical research and medical technology systems. A special problem faced by the biomedical research sector is the rapidly decreasing relative level of federal funding available (Rogers, 1996).

Health sciences knowledge and technology are put to use by the large number of people who work in the field, in the myriad professions and occupations that are found in it. The health sciences education system educates and trains the professionals and technicians who work in the health care system. In health care, *how* someone carries out a particular set of tasks and the nature of their motivation and attitude are sometimes as critical to success as *what* it is that they actually do. The health sciences education system plays a role in determining the character of the health care delivery system that goes beyond the mere technical and scientific content of the educational programs. (Medical education is touched on in chapter 2.)

Health Economics and Financing

As previously noted, in 1994 the United States spent close to $1 trillion on health services, more than 13% of its gross domestic product (Levit, 1996). Since the passage in 1965 of the Medicare legislation (providing for payment for certain health care services to persons 65 years of age and older and certain others covered by the Social Security System) inflation in health care costs has usually outstripped general inflation by a factor of two to three times, although during the 1990s the disparity between the two narrowed considerably (Levit, 1996, p. 207, Fig. 3).

Ultimately, all money paid for health services comes from the people. There are three major means by which money is transferred from them to the providers for the delivery of health services: (1) via government (in 1994 over 44% of total expenditures); (2) via insurance[2] and managed care companies (about 33% of the total); and (3) via direct payment (about 23% of the total, over 18% in direct out-of-pocket expenditures) (Levit, 1996). Government expenditures are both for services that it operates directly and services patients receive from independent providers. In this case government is a ''third-party payor'' (counting the patient as the first party and the provider, whether an individual or an institution, as the second).

The two major factors in the private insurance sector are Blue Cross/ Blue Shield (in most instances to date not for profit, although some are converting [Stocker, 1997]) and the commercial (for-profit) companies. With the growth of for-profit managed care, the commercial companies are becoming more of a factor in the private insurance sector. The major recipients of funds are the hospitals (36%), physicians (20%), pharmaceutical drug and ''other medical nondurables'' suppliers (8%), nursing homes (8%), dentists (4%), and government public health services (3%) (Levit, 1996, derived from Table 11).

The majority of health care personnel, for example nurses and other hospital employees, are paid by salary. Traditionally, private health care practitioners, such as physicians, dentists, chiropractors, and psychotherapists, have been paid on a fee-for-service basis. Under managed care an increasing number of this latter group of health professionals are receiving at least a portion of their incomes under a ''capitation'' payment system. In the past, U.S. health care institutions for the most part have operated either on a global budget or on some form of a cost-reimbursement basis. Again under managed care, a growing number of institutions too are receiving a ''capitated'' payment for each person they agree to provide

[2]The term *health insurance* is customarily applied to a system under which a company is paid money (a ''premium'') in advance for agreeing to pay for the costs (or some proportion of them) of a specified list of health services for a named beneficiary during a specified period of time. Under traditional health insurance, the care is not provided by the insurance company itself. Under managed care, the ''insurance'' and the care are either provided by the same company or the insurer and provider are very closely connected, usually by contract (see chapter 8).

The usage of the term ''health insurance'' is not in accordance with the usual meaning of the word ''insurance'': a group of individuals pay premiums to a financial entity to protect each member against the financial consequences of the occurrence of a *relatively rare* event, such as premature death or the loss of a dwelling to fire. The use of health services over a lifetime by any covered group of beneficiaries is not a rare event, however. Nevertheless, even though the usage is not strictly correct, we shall use the term ''health insurance,'' just as everyone else does.

services for, as needed by that person. (We cover financing mechanisms, expenditures, and methods of payment in some detail in chapters 5 and 8.)

Organizational Structure

Management of the Resources

If institutions, personnel, and financing are to be brought together in various settings in order to provide health care, they must be managed. System management includes four major activities: planning, administration, regulation, and evaluation. Each is closely related to the others. It should be noted that these terms are not used consistently in all the health care system sectors. A given action may be termed deliberate planning in one, normal administration in a second, and official regulation in a third. Too, the generic term ''management'' is often used interchangeably with the technically more narrow term ''administration.'' That should not be the case.

Planning

Planning may be defined as any deliberate action to determine unmet needs, set goals and objectives, design a program to meet them, and allocate resources for implementing the program in a systematic way. In this sense, health and health care planning in the United States and elsewhere can be said to have occurred with the establishment of the first hospital or the organization of the first governmental office of public health. Even though virtually all health care delivery entities engage in some form of health planning at some time or other, as customarily used, the term *health planning* refers to the actions of a governmental or quasi-governmental agency carrying out the functions just described. The results of the activity can be applied at any health care system level, from the local to the national.

In terms of backing up the findings and decisions of health care planning agencies in the U.S. with the force of law, health care planning in the United States has been very weak. It has been largely confined to hospital construction. In the mid-1990s in many parts of the U.S. there is no official planning function in place at all. Major decisions, even on such matters as medical school mergers, the growth of the managed care approach to the delivery of health services to the people, and the concomitant expansion of profit making in the health care field, with the exception of antitrust considerations, are being left to the institutional/provider parties themselves. (For a further discussion of health and health care planning, see chapter 7.)

Regulation

Somewhat paradoxically, in the U.S. health care system regulation is highly developed. Government regulation is primarily a reactive not a proactive process. Government regulation in the health care system usually occurs after, for example, serious financial problems have occurred or serious defects in quality are encountered. (There is also regulation in the public health sector, for example, in response to a corporate entity undertaking an activity that threatens the health, safety, or comfort of some significant group of people in the society.)

Because of the highly decentralized, primarily private, administrative structure and the absence of planning, many problems and abuses have developed in the system over time. In response, federal, state, and local governments from time to time have imposed health care system regulation in an attempt both to correct past problems and to prevent the development of new ones in the future. Presently, government regulation of the health care system operates at a modest level. Should the public find that the operations of the free market cannot meet all of their expressed needs, that level will likely rise again in the future.

Evaluation

Program evaluation *technique* is highly developed in the United States (Rossi & Freeman, 1993). A good deal of academic program evaluation is carried out. For a variety of public policy reasons, however, not the least of which is the absence of any national health system or national health planning system, actual applied program evaluation is often not done in the U.S. For example, in the mid-1990s managed care development was moving ahead swiftly with little evaluation of the effectiveness of the approach of the several different forms in meeting their own stated goals and objectives, much less objectively determined societal ones (Kodner, 1996).

(Neither program evaluation nor medical quality assessment is considered in this book. For an in-depth discussion of the latter, see chapter 14 in Kovner, A. & Jonas, S. (Eds.), 1996, *Jonas–Kovner Health Care Delivery in the United States* (6th ed.). New York: Springer Publishing Co., 1998.)

Administration

The administration of health services is a complex matter, itself the subject of many lengthy books (e.g., Shortell & Kaluzny, 1994, to which the reader is referred for an authoritative treatment of the subject). Although the *principles* of good administration and management apply equally, the many different types of health services organizations do face different types of administrative problems.

As an example, consider an administrative/management problem with which hospitals around the country are wrestling. Its resolution will require major changes in the way in which hospitals are structured. Those structural changes will in turn require major changes in the way people think and feel. With a few exceptions, hospitals are not used to mounting coordinated *programs*, but rather to delivering individual *services*, each component putting in its piece more or less as it sees fit. Most important, medical staff are used to functioning independently, not as part of a hospital team (Sanderson, 1996/1997).

Many of the present contradictions that are evident in the role and work of service, teaching, and research in hospitals will have to be resolved before these administrative problems can be solved. Managed care puts especial strains on the administration and management of hospitals, although the problems raised, respectively, by the for-profit and not-for-profit varieties are rather different. (See also chapter 3, Hospitals, chapter 7, Planning, and chapter 8, Managed Care.)

Health Services Program Auspices

The output of any health care delivery system is often described in terms of its major "health services programs." The forms and proportionate role of the auspice of each program differ among national systems. In the United States, as in most countries, there are five major types of health program auspices: the principal governmental health authorities, other agencies of government with health functions, the private health care sector, nonhealth care commercial enterprises with health functions, and voluntary health agencies. It is within each of the health services programs that the five elements of the system—facilities, personnel, commodities, knowledge, and money—interact to produce health services.

Government in Health Services

In the United States all three levels of government—federal, state, and local—directly operate certain health services programs, for example, the Federal Department of Veterans Affairs hospital system, the state mental hospitals, and the local government public hospitals. Furthermore, by being the conduit for almost half of the money paid for health services, collecting and disseminating information, educating and training personnel directly and providing financial support for many private health sciences educational institutions, being the largest player in the biomedical research arena, and operating the various public health services and regulatory functions, government is closely involved with virtually all health services programs.

The principal health agency of the U.S. federal government is the Department of Health and Human Services, headed by a Cabinet-level Secretary. It is responsible for the federal Social Security program, the (diminishing) federal role in the state-run public assistance programs, and the main federal programs in biomedical research, regulation, financing, and public health. Many of the Department's responsibilities are met by allocation of money and delegation of authority to other public and private entities throughout the nation that are concerned with health matters, of which there are many.

In each of the 50 states there is a major health agency. In some states it is combined with agencies for social welfare or other functions as at the federal level. The administrative configuration and scope of functions of the state health agencies are highly variable. The heads of these agencies are ordinarily appointed by the state's governor. Administratively they are responsible entirely to the governor and not at all to the U.S. Department of Health and Human Services. Only insofar as certain standards must be met as a condition for receipt of certain federal monies, must the state accept national direction.

Similarly, below the level of state government, there are units of local government—counties, cities, and occasionally special health services districts—that also have a major health agency. Most of these have great autonomy, although on certain health matters the local health department may carry out functions delegated by the state agency.

Finally, there are a variety of health-related functions that are carried by nonhealth government agencies. For example, at the federal level, the Department of Labor runs the Occupational Safety and Health Administration, and the Department of Agriculture sets national nutrition standards in cooperation with the Department of Health and Human Services. At all three levels of government, environmental protection services are often provided by an independent agency, for example, the Environmental Protection Administration at the federal level. (For a closer look at government activities in health care delivery see chapters 5 and 7.)

Voluntary Agencies

In all countries there are nongovernmental agencies that play a role in health care systems. They are commonly known as "voluntary agencies." In the United States the group includes, for example, the American Heart

Association, the American Cancer Society, and the Visiting Nurse Association. Voluntary health agencies have a wide variety of functions: to perform a service not rendered by other agencies, to pursue certain research or service objectives with special vigor and dedication, to advance or protect the interests of a certain population group, to engage in public and political education and advocacy, to carry out certain tasks at the behest of official bodies.

Like any corporation, in order to stay in business they must take in more money than they spend. In the voluntary agency, however, the excess of income over expenses does not accrue to any individual(s) but rather supports the expansion of the agency's work. These corporations are thus alternatively termed "not for profit" or "nonprofit." The voluntary agency may be devoted exclusively to health purposes, or health services may be incidental to certain larger purposes, such as those of church groups or religious missions (domestic or foreign).

A subset of the voluntary health agency is the health professional organization, for example, the American Medical Association, the American Nurses Association, the American College of Preventive Medicine, the American Medical Athletics Association. They are financed by membership dues, journal subscriptions and advertising fees, and on occasion research grants and contracts. They are primarily concerned with, for example, advancing the perceived professional and economic interests of their members, through public education, continuing professional education, litigation, legislative and political action, and, on occasion, tradeunionlike activity. As well, they may also focus on advancing scientific knowledge and understanding, setting and maintaining professional standards, and educating the public about health and disease.

For-Profit Enterprises with Health Functions

There are two classes of for-profit enterprises that provide health services: commercial entities that provide health services to the public, and corporations which deliver health services to their employees.

For-Profit or "Proprietary" Health Service Enterprises. These play an increasingly significant role in the U.S. health care system. There are five groups. First are those engaged in "commodities production," mentioned above. Second, nursing homes for the aged and chronically ill have long been predominately proprietary, with about 80% of their beds in units operated for profit. Third, are the for-profit general hospitals, both part of managed care companies and independent. They house about 11% of the nonfederal short-term hospital beds in the country (*Health,*

1996, Table 107). Fourth are the commercial health insurance companies (see chapter 5) as well as those insurance companies providing professional liability (malpractice) coverage. Fifth is the rapidly growing for-profit managed care sector that itself has developed from three different streams: the proprietary hospital sector, the commercial health insurance sector, and *de novo* (see chapter 8).

Employee Health. In the United States, in-plant employee health services are generally of circumscribed scope, except in large establishments (more than 500 workers). In smaller factories, they are usually limited to the provision of first aid by an industrial nurse or perhaps only a medicine chest for self-use. Large plants or mines may maintain a staff of physicians and nurses that performs periodic and preplacement examinations, treats any work-related illnesses, disabilities, or injuries, and may engage in worksite wellness activities (O'Donnell & Harris, 1994).

Enterprises in isolated locations, such as railroad junctions or lumber mills, may operate comprehensive medical care programs. Industrial firms are obligated by law to protect workers from accidents and occupational diseases, although enforcement, carried out by the Federal Occupational and Health Administration and in certain states designated state agencies, is often weak.

Private Professional Practice

The U.S. health care delivery system has traditionally been dominated by private medical and other health professional practice. As of the mid-1990s, though as noted on a number of previous occasions system trends have begun changing many of these relationships, office and in-hospital medical care (both general and specialized), dental care, chiropractic, pharmacy, optical, medical and nonmedical psychotherapeutic, speech and audiology services, the fitting of prosthetic appliances, as well as others, are still furnished primarily by private practitioners.

It is especially noteworthy that, even when the financial support for health services has been collectivized, as in the various public or private health insurance programs and managed care, the direct provision of health services has remained substantially in the market created by individual practitioners. In private medical practice, for example, whether it is carried out in the physician's office or a hospital, the service is rendered by an individual physician to a private patient of that physician. The responsible third-party payor, if any, pays a private fee to the provider. (For a further discussion of private medical practice, see chapter 2.)

Thus true medical group practice or multidisciplinary team practice are still relatively rare in the United States (see chapter 8). However, one of the intriguing aspects of managed care is that private practicing physicians who formerly (informally) contracted directly with their patients are now in one sense becoming collectivized as well, as previously noted. Under managed care the service contract is between the managed care company and the patient. The physician also contracts with the company (not the patient) to provide care for a set of patients. And increasingly, the physician is no longer paid on a piecemeal, fee-for-service basis but rather a fee-for-total-care basis for each patient under his or her care (called "capitation").

THE DELIVERY OF HEALTH SERVICES

Several components of the health care system work together to produce health services for individuals ("personal health services") and population groups ("community health services").[3] To distinguish the personal from the other parts of the system, what happens in the former is customarily called the "delivery of health services." These services are usually further categorized, as primary, secondary, or tertiary.

Primary Care

In functional terms, primary care is the care that most people need most of the time for most of their health concerns (see also chapter 4). Primary care includes a wide range of personal preventive and treatment measures. In the industrialized countries these measures are usually provided by a physician, although in some parts of the United States nurse practitioners and physicians' assistants are also being employed to provide primary care.

Common forms of personal preventive measures are the promotion of personal lifestyle/behavior change (e.g., smoking cessation), immunization, prenatal care, and periodic health examination for early disease detection. Primary care treatment covers most health services given to patients who are not in institutional beds, although there is some overlap in both directions. (Primary care is discussed in more detail in chapter 4.)

[3] A personal health service is one given directly to an individual, for example, treatment for an upper respiratory infection, or the setting and casting of a fractured ankle. The recipient is almost invariably aware that he/she is receiving the service. A community health service is one provided to a group of people as a group. Each group member may be aware that he or she is receiving the service, for example, public health education on smoking cessation, but often the group member is unaware of the service received, for example, as in the provision of pure water supply and sanitary sewage disposal.

Secondary and Tertiary Care

Tertiary care, which is at the other end of the spectrum from primary care, consists of the highly specialized diagnostic, therapeutic, and rehabilitative services, requiring staff and equipment "that transcend the capabilities of the average community hospital" (Rogatz, 1970, p. 47). Such care, available largely at major medical centers, includes, for instance, transplant and open-heart surgery and other technologically complex procedures, complex chemo- and radiotherapy for cancer, and the preservation of very low-birth-weight premature infants.

Secondary care, the most difficult level to define, includes services that are available both in community hospitals and physicians' offices. Ideally they are arranged through referral or consultation after a preliminary evaluation by a primary-care practitioner. Secondary services include most surgery and the services of such specialists as diagnostic radiologists, cardiologists, and endocrinologists.

In the U.S., both secondary and tertiary health care services are highly developed. That development has not always occurred in response to a well-documented need or in a planned way so as to make for the most efficient use of scarce resources.

Care of Special Populations and Disorders

In all health care systems there are special programs providing primary, secondary, and tertiary care for certain population groups that are defined by age, gender, or occupation, and for the control of certain specific health disorders. In the U.S. many of the special programs are provided by government, such as those for military personnel and dependents, military service veterans, and Native Americans. Other populations for which special programs of health care have been created include: railroad workers, migrant farm workers, certain industrial workers, school children, college and university students.

Special programs can also be organized by type of illness. Mental illness is the most important health disorder for which special subsystems of health care delivery are organized in the United States. Hospitalization for mental illness takes place primarily in special mental hospitals, primarily financed and operated by state governments (although the state hospital system has been drastically shrunk since the mid-1960s and community hospitals equipped to treat these individuals increasingly have been admitting short-term patients with psychiatric diagnoses).

Ambulatory care for mental illness and emotional problems can be provided in private practice by psychiatrists, clinical psychologists, psychiatric social workers, and other therapists. There are also several thousand public or voluntary mental health clinics serving primarily low-income patients. A national community mental health center system, which was promised back in the 1960s, to functionally replace the state mental hospital system has never been built, however.

Tuberculosis (TB), before the steep decline in its incidence and prevalence that occurred after the discovery of effective antibiotics for it at mid-century, also warranted a special network of clinics and hospitals (sanitaria) for its detection and care. (The current acquired immunodeficiency syndrome (AIDS)-related increase in the incidence of tuberculosis, although a serious problem, is not of a magnitude that will lead to the reestablishment of anything like the TB hospital system.)

PROBLEMS IN HEALTH CARE DELIVERY IN THE UNITED STATES

For all of its resources, personnel, facilities, skills, knowledge, money, and ability to do wondrous things to and with the human body, the U.S. health care delivery is plagued with problems. Some observers call the situation a "crisis." "Sudden worsening" is part of the definition of "crisis," however, and most of the observed problems have been with us for a very long time. Thus it can be fairly stated that the health care delivery system is *not* in crisis, but rather that it has serious problems of long-standing, some of which are seemingly intractable.

It is fascinating that for the most part these problems are not those of a technical and/or scientific inability to deal with diseases or other health deficits. Nor is the problem one of lack of money, as it is in so many other countries. In the U.S., the principal problems are as follows:

- We spend too *much*, not too *little*.
- The rate of rise in costs, although it has moderated in the 1990s, has been for the most part uncontrollable by any interventions tried to date.
- The geographic and demographic distribution of health services is highly variable.
- Much that could be done to prevent disease and promote health using available knowledge and techniques is not done.
- There are serious misallocations both by type of health care institutions and personnel.
- Many health care needs are undermet (e.g., not enough home health care for the infirm elderly), whereas others are overmet (e.g., too many hospital beds, too much surgery, too much diagnostic testing).

In short, the problems are not those of lack of resources, but rather of their misuse and misallocation. As far back as 1932, the findings of the first comprehensive study of health care delivery in the United States were summarized in these terms (Committee on the Costs of Medical Care, 1970, p. 2):

> The problem of providing satisfactory medical service to all the people of the United States at costs which they can meet is a pressing one. At the present time, many persons do not receive service which is adequate either in quantity or quality, and the costs of service are inequably distributed. The result is a tremendous amount of preventable physical pain and mental anguish, needless deaths, economic inefficiency, and social waste. Furthermore, these conditions are, as the following pages will show, largely unnecessary. The United States has the economic resources, the organizing ability, and the technical experience to solve this problem.

The committee, chaired by Ray Lyman Wilbur, a past president of the American Medical Association, had been created in 1927 to look into problems of the health care system. Strikingly, some would say unfortunately, the statement is entirely applicable over 70 years later.

In the 1960s and 1970s, observers of the U.S. health care system, of differing political persuasions, often spoke of ''crisis.'' Indeed there has been a long line of critical reports and studies going back many years. (For an introductory bibliography of such reports, see Appendix I.)

In 1970, the editors of *Fortune Magazine*, eerily echoing the paragraph quoted from the CCMC *Final Report* wrote (p. 9):

> American medicine, the pride of the nation for many years, stands now on the brink of chaos. To be sure, our medical practitioners have their great moments of drama and triumph. But much of the U.S. medical care, particularly the everyday business of preventing and treating routine illnesses, is inferior in quality, wastefully dispensed, and inequitably financed. Medical manpower and facilities are so maldistributed that large segments of the population, especially the urban poor and those in rural areas, get virtually no care at all even though their illnesses are most numerous and, in a medical sense, often easy to cure.

Also in an echo of the CCMC *Final Report*, and eerily presaging the problems of our own time, none other than President Richard M. Nixon said in 1971 that:

> For a growing number of Americans, the cost of care is becoming prohibitive. Even those who can afford most care may find themselves impover-

ished by a catastrophic medical expenditure. The quality of medicine varies widely with geography and income. Because we pay so little attention to preventing disease and treating it early, too many people get sick and need intensive treatment. Costs have skyrocketed but values have not kept pace. We are investing more of our nation's resources in the health of our people, but we are not getting a full return on our investment (Nixon, 1994, p. 11).

In 1973, the Research and Policy Committee of the Committee for Economic Development, with a board composed of representatives of many of the leading American corporations and banks, came to the following conclusions concerning the system (p. 17):

First, faulty allocation of resources is a major cause of inadequacies and inequalities in U.S. health services that result today in poor or substandard care for large segments of the population. Second, the task of assuring all people the ability to cope financially with the costs of health care has been made realizable by the substantial base of coverage now provided by both private and public insurance plans. Third, unless step-by-step alterations are made in the means of delivering services and paying providers, closing the gaps in financing would overburden an inadequate system and offer little prospect of materially improving the quality and quantity of medical services of the health of the American people.

Moving to our own time, in 1990 perhaps the most prominent of a spate of reports and program proposals for health care delivery reform issued that year had this to say (Pepper Commission, p. 2):

The American health care system is approaching a breaking point. Rapidly rising medical costs are increasing the numbers of people without health coverage and straining the system's capacity to provide care for those who cannot pay. The gap is widening between the majority of Americans, who can take advantage of the best medical services in the world, and the rest, who find it hard to get even basic needed care. As the gap increases, the weight of financing care for those without adequate coverage is undermining the stability of our health care institutions. Even for the majority, the explosive growth in health care costs is steadily eroding the private insurance system—the bulwark they count on as their defense against financial risk in case of illness.

Finally, in introducing his ill-fated Health Security Act in 1993 (see chapter 9), President William J. Clinton had this to say (DPC, 1993, p. iii):

Americans are blessed with the world's finest doctors and nurses, the best hospitals, the most advanced medical technology, and the most promising

> research on the face of the earth. We cherish—and we will never surrender—our right to choose who treats us and how we get our care.
>
> But today our health care system is badly broken.
>
> Insurance has become a contest of finding only the healthiest people to cover. Millions of Americans are just a pink slip away from losing their health coverage, one serious illness away from losing their savings. Millions more are locked into jobs for fear of losing their benefits. And small business owners throughout our nation want to provide health care for their employees and families but can't get it or can't afford it.
>
> Next year we will spend more than one trillion dollars on health care—and still leave 37 million Americans without health insurance, and 25 million more with inadequate coverage. . . . In short, all the things that are wrong with our health care system threaten everything's that right.

THE PRESENT SITUATION

In the mid-1990s the situation was about the same. Costs continued to rise, although perhaps not at the same precipitous rate that had been experienced in the 1980s. An ever-increasing number of persons had no health insurance and for many of them that fact created serious family financial difficulties (Donelan et al., 1996). Hospital beds were still maldistributed, with an oversupply of beds in voluntary and proprietary hospitals in many parts of the country and undersupply of beds in public general hospitals in most cities. There was a problem too with physician oversupply in many of the specialties, although there was still and undersupply of primary-care physicians (Rivo et al., 1995).

Rationing of health services by race, age, and geography had become a major concern (Geiger, 1996). There were deficiencies in the quality of medical care, as well as in the measures designed to control quality (IOM, 1990). There was a continuing tendency, particularly among teaching-hospital-based physicians, to stress the unusual at the expense of the commonplace, to focus on patients with acute physical problems at the expense of patients who are chronically ill or have mental problems, and to emphasize treatment rather than prevention (Jonas, 1988).

As demonstrated by the quotes presented above, few, if any, of these problems with our health care system are new. Over time they have simply undergone gradual changes in size and relative importance. Indeed, certain of the major problems considered important by the Committee on the Costs of Medical Care that are still pressing today originated in our country and those of our European forebears in the 17th, 18th, and 19th centuries (Freymann, 1974). The problems are not only of long-standing. They are embedded in the whole fabric of American society.

The fundamental conundrum facing health policy analysts, political leaders who would like to change things, and above all the American people is: "How come the findings and recommendations of a major report on health care issued in 1932 and echoed strongly for over 60 years have never been acted upon? How come things haven't changed?" Finding and framing the answer(s) to that riddle is not the function of this book. But perhaps some of the information contained in this volume will enable readers to find the correct answer(s) for themselves. For those inclined, armed with that understanding, they may be able to proceed to do something about the situation.

REFERENCES

Adams, P. F., & Marano, M. A. Current estimates from the National Health Interview Survey, 1994. *Vital and Health Statistics*, Series 10, No. 193, December, 1995.

Adler, N. E. et al. Socioeconomic inequities in health. *Journal of the American Medical Association, 269,* 3140, 1993.

AHA (American Hospital Association). *AHA Guide to the Health Care Field, 1995–96.* Chicago: 1995.

Committee on the Costs of Medical Care. *Medical care for the American people.* Chicago: University of Chicago Press, 1932. Reprinted, Washington, DC: USDHEW, 1970.

Consumer Reports. Can HMOs help solve the health-care crisis? October 1996, p. 28.

DPC (Domestic Policy Council). *Health security: The president's report to the American people.* Washington, DC: The White House, October 1993.

Donelan, K., et al. Whatever happened to the health insurance crisis in the United States? *Journal of the American Medical Association, 276,* 1346, 1996.

Fortune Magazine Editors. *Our ailing medical system: It's time to operate.* New York: Harper & Row, 1970.

Fubini, S. Not-for-profit vs. for-profit—Reading the tea leaves. *Health Care Trends Report, 10*(4), 1996, p. 1.

Freymann, J. G. *The American health care system: Its genesis and trajectory.* New York: Medcom Press, 1974.

Geiger, J. Race and health care—An American dilemma? *New England Journal of Medicine, 335,* 815, 1996.

Ginzberg, E. The health care market. *Journal of the American Medical Association, 276,* 777, 1996.

Grove, R. D., & Hetzel, A. M. *Vital statistics rates in the United States: 1940–1960.* Washington, DC: National Center for Health Statistics, USDHEW, 1968.

IOM (Institute of Medicine). Lohr, K. N. (Ed.). *Medicare: A strategy for quality assurance* (Vols. 1 & 2). Washington, DC: National Academy Press, 1990.

Jonas, S. Health promotion in medical education. *American Journal of Health Promotion, 3,* 37, 1988.

Kassirer, J. P. Managed care and the morality of the marketplace. *New England Journal of Medicine, 333,* 50, 1995.

Kodner, D. Managed care. (a course) New York University, September–December, 1996.

KPMG (KPMG Peat Marwick LLP). The impact of managed care on U.S. markets. Executive Summary, Costa Mesa, CA, 1996.

Lehman, L. B. Health of the public: The private-sector challenge (letter). *Journal of the American Medical Association, 276,* 1951, 1996.

Levit, K. R., et al. HCFA (Health Care Financing Administration). National health expenditures, 1994. *Health Care Financing Review, 17*(3), 205, 1996.

McGinniss, J. M., & Foege, W. H. Actual causes of death in the United States. *Journal of the American Medical Association, 270,* 2207, 1993.

Nixon, R. M. Message to Congress on health insurance. Washington, DC, February 18, 1971, reprinted in *The New Republic*, Sept. 19 & 26, 1994, p. 11.

O'Donnell, M. P. & Harris, J. S. *Health promotion in the workplace.* Albany, NY: Delmar, 1994.

Pappas, G., et al. The increasing disparity in mortality between socioeconomic groups in the United States, 1960 and 1986. *New England Journal of Medicine, 329,* 103, 1993.

Pepper Commission. *A call for action.* Executive Summary, Washington, DC: U.S. Government Printing Office, September 1990.

Research and Policy Committee. *Building a national health-care system.* New York: Committee for Economic Development, 1973.

Rivo, M. L., et al. Managed health care: Implications for the physician workforce and medical education. *Journal of the American Medical Association, 274,* 712, 1995.

Roemer, M. *National health systems of the world* (Vol. I). New York: Oxford University Press, 1991.

Roemer, M. *National health systems of the world* (Vol. II). New York: Oxford University Press, 1993.

Rogatz, P. The health care system: Planning. *Hospitals*, April 16, 1970, p. 47.

Rogers, P. New politics in science. *Science, 274,* 1445, 1996.

Rossi, P. H., & Freeman, H. E. *Evaluation: A systematic approach.* Newbury Park, CA: Sage Publications, 1993.

Sanderson, S. C. Collaboration and team-building are critical skills for up-and-coming faculty. *AAMC Reporter, 6*(4), 1996/1997.

Schwartz, E., et al. Black/white comparisons of deaths preventable by medical interventions. *International Journal of Epidemiology, 19,* 591, 1990.

Sherill, R. The madness of the market. *The Nation*, Jan. 9/16, p. 45, 1995.

Shortell, S. M., & Kaluzny, A. D. *Health care management.* Albany, NY: Delmar, 1994.

Singh, G. K., et al. Advance report of final mortality statistics, 1994. *Monthly Vital Statistics Report (MVSR), 45*(3), Suppl. Sept. 30, 1996.

Stocker, M. A. What is Empire proposing and why? Presented at *New York Academy of Medicine*, February 14, 1997.

Thurow, L. C. Companies merge; Families break up. *New York Times*, Sept. 3, 1995.

Wennberg, J., et al. *The Dartmouth atlas of health care.* Chicago: American Hospital Publishing, 1996.

Chapter 2
Personnel

OVERVIEW[1]

In 1994 almost 10.6 million people, about 8.6% of all persons employed in the United States, were working in the health care industry. Close to half of them worked in hospitals, 16% in nursing and personal care facilities, and over 13% in physicians' offices (*Health*, 1996, Table 96). These percentages had changed only marginally since 1988. Altogether, the U.S. Department of Labor has identified about 700 categories of skilled health occupations. Among the health care professionals, in 1993 there were about 1,950,000 active registered nurses, close to 600,000 active allopathic (M.D. degree) physicians, and over 32,000 osteopathic (D.O. degree) physicians, 172,000 pharmacists, 154,000 dentists, 28,000 optometrists, and 13,000 podiatrists (*Health*, 1996, Table 101).

In 1993, in the community hospitals alone (see chapter 3 for definition) there were close to 35,000 dieticians, over 40,000 physical therapists and aides, and over 25,000 medical social workers (*Health*, 1996, Table 102). Also in the community hospitals that year there were about 760,000 licensed practical nurses, more than 165,000 laboratory personnel, close to 120,000 radiologic service personnel, and about 65,000 respiratory therapists and technicians.

The ratio of other health personnel to physicians reflects the complexity of the U.S. health care system. In 1993, when as noted there were about 630,000 physicians (M.D. and D.O.) in active practice, there were almost 16 other health care workers for each physician. (In 1988, there were close to 18 other health care workers for each physician. The drop may be due in part to certain changes in the method of counting the numbers

[1]Except as otherwise noted, the data used in this chapter, variously for 1993 and 1994, are taken from *Health United States, 1995*, National Center for Health Statistics, Hyattsville, MD: DHHS Pub. No. (PHS) 96-1232, May 1996.

in the various health worker categories.) This compares with about three other health care workers per doctor in 1920 (Donabedian et al., 1980). Most of these "other personnel" have skills learned through special training. Only about one fifth are nonspecific clerical, custodial, or similar personnel.

Under the laws of most states, only physicians, dentists, and a relatively few other types of practitioner may serve patients directly, without the authorization of another health professional licensed for independent practice. Among the other independent health professions are: chiropractic, optometry, podiatry, psychotherapy, and, in some states, midwifery and physical therapy. For the most part, nurses work on the orders of physicians, although in certain circumstances, in certain states, some nurses called "nurse practitioners" (see below) can work independently.

Other types of health care providers working on the orders and under at least the general supervision of physicians include: clinical laboratory, x-ray, electrocardiographic, and other specialized technicians such as those who operate kidney dialysis machines; in rehabilitation services there are physical, occupational, and speech therapists; in dental care one finds dental hygienists, dental technicians, and dental assistants. Nutritionists and dietitians, statisticians and statistical clerks, medical record librarians and information system specialists, cardiorespiratory therapists, audiologists, and orthopedic technicians perform other special tasks.

Many of these occupations originally developed out of the nursing profession. In countries less developed than the United States, work done in the United States by a laboratory technician, physical therapist, or dietitian is often done by a nurse. But in the industrialized countries, the diversification and specialization that occurred in medicine as medical science and technology advanced and became more complex also has taken place in the nursing profession. Consider, for example, the development of the operating-room nurse, the intensive-care nurse, and the nurse anesthetist. In the next two sections we consider the two largest health professions, medicine and nursing, in some more detail.

PHYSICIANS

Licensure

According to the Medical Practice Act of New York State (Article 131, Para. 6521 of the State Education Law) (USNY [Medicine], 1995, p. 31): "The practice of the profession of medicine is . . . diagnosing, treating, operating or prescribing for any human disease, pain, injury, deformity or physical condition.'' In the U.S., the medical license is granted by the states. To qualify for a medical license in New York State, for example, one must (USNY [Medicine], 1995): hold an M.D. or D.O. degree or its equivalent from a school meeting the state education department's requirements, have certain postgraduate (''residency'') practice experience, pass a medical licensure examination as designated by the department, be a citizen or resident alien, be of ''good moral character,'' and pay a fee. (All states have similar requirements.) In practice in the 1990s, few medical-school graduates entered practice before completing at least 3 more years of residency training.

Some Basic Data

As of 1994, about 88% of the 684,000 living, presently or formerly licensed, U.S. allopathic doctors of medicine (M.D.s) were in active practice (*Health*, 1996, Table 99).[2] About 23% of the 605,000 active M.D.s received their medical training outside of the U.S. and Canada. That is quite a remarkable percentage considering the size and the ongoing investment of the U.S. medical education system (see below). But as Fitzhugh Mullan (1995) has pointed out, despite the output of the U.S. medical schools, physician manpower needs in many medically underserved areas could not be met without a steady influx of so-called ''international medical graduates'' to U.S. residency programs,especially those in hospitals situated in those same underserved areas.

Over 22,000 of the active physicians were in federal government service, most of them in the armed forces or units what was formerly the U.S. Public Health Service (see chapter 6). About 85% of the federal physicians worked in patient-care services. These percentages had varied marginally since 1988. In 1994, about 538,000 (over 92%) of all nonfederal physicians worked in patient care. Of those, about 75% were in office-based practice, about 15% were house staff (residents in training), and almost 8% were fully qualified physicians working full time in hospitals (*Health*, 1996, Table 99).

The close to 45,000 nonfederal professionally active physicians who were not in patient care (a slight decrease from 1992) worked in administration, medical education, research, state and local health services, the pharmaceutical industry, and the like. Among the several medical specialties, the largest numbers were found in internal medicine, about 65,000; general and family practice, about 58,000; pediatrics, close to 31,000;

[2]Please note that there are some unexplained inconsistencies between the several tables in *Health, U.S. 1995* reporting physician supply.

obstetrics and gynecology, close to 28,000; and general surgery, over 24,000.

In 1994, the overall M.D. and D.O. physician:population ratio was 23.5 per 10,000 (*Health*, 1996, Table 97). This is up from a post-World War II low in 1960 of 14 and from the 1988 figure of 22.6 per 10,000. A wide variation existed by geographic region. The highest ratio, 28 per 10,000, was found in New England, whereas the lowest, 16.7, was found in the West South Central (Arkansas, Oklahoma, Texas, and Louisiana). By state, the ratio ranged from a low of 12.4 in Mississippi to a high of 32 in Massachusetts.

Although there are no known differences in health status that vary consistently with physician/population ratios, utilization of health services is generally higher in those areas that have more physicians (Eisenberg, 1986; Leape et al., 1989; Wennberg, 1984, 1996). Among the factors influencing the amount of work physicians do are income goals, desired practice style, personal characteristics, practice setting, and standards established by clinical leadership (Eisenberg, 1986).

Private Medical Practice

The primary mode of organization of physicians in the United States (and indeed of most the other health care providers who are licensed to practice independently) has been what is called ''private practice.'' Traditionally, the private practitioner contracts directly with patients (although almost never in writing) to provide a set of services in return for payment of a fee by the patient directly or, more commonly, a ''third-party payor'' (such as a health insurance company or the Medicare program). This arrangement is appropriately enough called the *fee-for-service* system.

A combination of the licensing laws of the state in which the physician is located, the requirements of the malpractice insurer, and the stipulations of the hospital to which the physician admits patients if he/she is a hospital-staff member, regulate what each physician in private practice may do to and for patients.

In the era of managed care, this mode of physician organization is changing (Bodenheimer & Grumbach, 1994). It is, however, difficult to get accurate data on how many physicians are working in which kind of contract and payment arrangements, and thus keep up with the quickly changing picture. In 1989 about three quarters of all physicians in active practice, including hospital-based physicians but excluding house staff, were in private practice (Gillis & Wilke, 1989). By 1994 that proportion had fallen to about two thirds (AMA, 1996).

Over time the proportion of physicians working on salary has increased, especially among younger physicians. Among the reasons are the attractiveness of a regular salary and a comprehensive fringe-benefit package; the provision of medical malpractice insurance by the employer; regular hours and regular night and weekend coverage schedules; the difficulty of entering into private practice in many desirable living areas, many of which have a physician excess; the high costs of starting a private practice, a particular burden to so many of today's new physicians who enter professional life with a large debt accumulated in the course of their medical education; and finally, avoidance of the trials and tribulations of office practice with a managed care company looking over one's shoulder (see chapter 8).

Patterns of Practice

An important feature of medical-practice organization in the U.S. is that most physicians see patients both on an ambulatory basis in their own offices and as hospital inpatients. (A small percentage of doctors do not have hospital appointments. How many is not known. Most of them are probably in urban areas.) In most other countries, physicians either see ambulatory patients only or work full time in hospitals (see below).

The unusual American arrangement offers some significant advantages to the patient. For the many conditions for which one physician is technically competent to provide both ambulatory and inpatient care there is continuity of care. In many cases requiring surgery, the nonsurgical referring physician will participate in the pre- and postoperative phases of care in the hospital.

With the advent of managed care, however, this picture may be changing, along with many others. Managed care emphasizes the use of the primary-care physician. Most plans do not allow beneficiaries to see a specialist without seeing, or at least receiving the approval of, their primary-care physician first.

The primary-care physician has two main functions under managed care. One function is to provide most of the health care that his or her patients need most of the time while coordinating the rest as a "gatekeeper" for what is best for the *patient* (see also chapter 4). The other is to act as the "gatekeeper" for the *system*, controlling the use of hospital and specialist care, at least as much for fiscal as for medical reasons (see chapter 8). This could lead to a pattern modeled on the British system. In Great Britain the primary physicians, called general practitioners, see patients almost exclusively on an ambulatory basis. The specialists, although seeing patients on both an ambulatory and inpatient basis, are virtually the only ones who handle hospitalized patients.

As two observers noted (Wachter & Goldman, 1996, p. 514):

> [Taking into account] the realities of managed care [in the U.S.] and its emphasis on efficiency . . . we anticipate the rapid growth of a new breed of physicians we call ''hospitalists''—specialists in in-patient medicine—who will be responsible for managing the care of hospitalized patients in the same way that primary care physicians are responsible for managing the care of outpatients.

Medical Specialization[3]

Specialization is a prominent feature of American medical practice. The explosion of biomedical knowledge and technology that began early in this century has made it ever more difficult, in the areas of complex pathophysiological states and complicated surgery, for a physician to master in depth more than one small piece of what biomedical science and practice can do.

In contrast to the depth of knowledge and skill required in the high-tech specialties, the specialties of family medicine, primary-care pediatrics, and primary-care internal medicine demand a great breadth of knowledge and competency. In contrast, in many of the non-primary care specialties, even though considerable depth of knowledge and skill is required, since they are in a relatively narrow range, the practice of medicine is often easier for the physician than it is in primary care.

The knowledge–technology explosion is only one factor that accounts for the ever-increasing specialization of American medicine. Another factor is the financial incentive involved in specialization: almost always there has been more money to be made in the specialties than in primary care. And, there has never been a health manpower planning policy in this country (see chapter 7).

Specialization has its advantages for patients. Specialists do develop a high degree of knowledge and, if necessary, skill in dealing with their areas of expertise, which is very beneficial to the patient. But it also has its disadvantages. Specialists tend to concentrate on a particular organ or organ system to the exclusion of the others. The patient's overall well-being may suffer if there is no professional in the picture who can (1)

---

[3]A particularly erudite and detailed history of the development of specialization in American medical practice is presented by Rosemary Stevens in her still relevant history, *American medicine and the public interest*, New Haven, CT: Yale University Press, 1971.

see the patient as a whole person; (2) put together into one clinical picture observations derived from a variety of patient complaints arising from different organ systems; (3) guide the patient through an intelligent utilization of the knowledge of several specialists; and (4) set up an organized means for communication among specialists.

This is not an argument against specialization per se; the vast expansion of medical knowledge requires such specialization, at least for a certain proportion of the profession. It is an argument for a more rational approach to the organization of specialists and a significant improvement in the provision of primary-care physician services (Colwill, 1986; Geyman, 1986; Relman, 1978; White, 1973).

In the mid-90s, with the advent of managed care the situation was beginning to change. Rivo et al. (1995, p. 712) presented the findings of the Sixth Report of the Congressional authorized Council on Graduate Medical Education (COGME):

1. Managed care has grown rapidly in both the private and public sectors and in most geographic areas; the rate of growth is likely to continue or accelerate in the future.
2. The growth in managed care will magnify physician workforce concerns expressed by COGME in prior reports. *Specifically, there is a large and growing oversupply of specialist and subspecialist physicians, and there is a modest need for more generalist physicians* [emphasis added].
3. Changes in the health care environment that have led to the growth in managed care will also have major effects on the allopathic and osteopathic medical education systems and their teaching institutions. These changes will likely result in decreased financial support for medical education at both the undergraduate and graduate levels, which could affect the quality of these endeavors.
4. The growth of managed care will magnify the deficiencies of the current educational system, yet will also provide new and essential educational opportunities to improve physicians' training for their future role.
5. Currently, there are many barriers and few incentives by which medical schools, residency programs, teaching hospitals, and managed care organizations can address problems related to the physician workforce and medical education priorities.

   In reference to the physician over-supply problem, COGME's estimated physician staffing requirement is 85 to 105 specialists per 100,000 population, which translates into a surplus of 125,000 specialists by the year 2000 and 170,000 by the year 2010, compared with

> the midpoint of the requirements range. During the same period, the generalist physician supply is projected to remain stable at 63 to 67 generalist physicians per 100,000 population, compared with the COGME'S estimated staffing requirements of 60 to 80 generalist physicians per 100,000 population. Compared with the midpoint, this represents a modest shortage of 20,000 generalist physicians in the year 2000, declining to 8000 (or near balance) in 2010.

Obviously, there were serious problems with both physician supply and medical education, indicating that a national planning effort of some kind was in order. But neither one of two major reports that appeared in 1996 addressing the issues raised by COGME made such a recommendation (IOM, 1996; PHPC, 1995). No, we were told, the "free market," perhaps with a bit of governmental nudging around the edges, would sort things out just fine (see also chapter 7).

Medical Education[4]

In the United States as of 1995, there were 125 fully accredited medical schools offering the M.D. degree and 16 offering the D.O. degree. Allopathic (M.D.) medical schools in the United States and Canada are accredited by a voluntary agency called the Liaison Committee on Medical Education. This agency is comprised of representatives from the American Medical Association and the Association of American Medical Colleges and their Canadian counterparts. Osteopathic (D.O.) medical schools are accredited by the American Osteopathic Association.

All but a few medical schools are attached to a university. In the university, the medical school is invariably a separate college with its own Dean (or the equivalent), sometimes loosely linked with other health professional schools in a "Health Sciences Center." About 60% of the medical schools are sponsored by state governments, as part of state public universities, while the rest are under private auspices. All the schools, however, have received substantial, although primarily indirect, financial support from the federal government for many years.

Entry to U.S. medical schools usually requires a bachelor's degree (requiring 4 years of study). The standard medical school program lasts another 4 years. It is customarily called "undergraduate medical education" even though in the university sense it is graduate education. This

[4]The data for this section on medical education are drawn from the "Medical Education/Pulse," American Medical Association, *Journal of the American Medical Association, 276,* pp. 659–758, 1996, unless otherwise noted.

is because in medical training the postmedical degree hospital-based residency experience is called "graduate medical education."

Although recently there have been some significant changes in the undergraduate medical education programs in perhaps a quarter of the U.S. medical schools (Ross & Feinberg, 1996), with more schools participating in the change process each year, a significant number of schools still employed what has been the standard curriculum since the early part of this century: 2 years of didactic basic science study followed by 2 years of clinical study with patients.

Admission to medical schools is selective (Barzansky et al., 1996). For the class entering 1995, there were about 46,600 applicants (up from 27,000 for the class of 1990) of whom about 17,300 found places. The ratio of applicants to places had been falling steadily through the 1980s from a high of 2.8 in 1973–1975. It was 1.6 in 1990. But by 1995 it had once again reached 2.7. The proportion of women in medical school has been increasing steadily since the early 1970s. In 1995 women accounted for 43% of the number of applicants, 43% of the entering class, and 41% of the graduating class that entered 4 years before.

Although the record for improving the admission rates for African Americans does not match that for women, some gains have been made in recent years. From the 1970s through 1990 the percentage of African American admissions remained unchanged at about 6%. By 1995 this number had increased to 9%. At the same time Latino admissions have increased moderately, as have those for Native Americans (by 1995, close to 1%). In 1995 Asian Americans accounted for close to one-quarter of all admissions.

The ratio of full-time faculty to students is very high, much higher than in virtually any other branch of education. In fact, in medical education the number of faculty actually *exceeds* the number of students by a ratio of 1.4:1. This is one of the reasons medical education is so expensive (Krakower et al., 1996). In 1994–1995, the medical schools collectively spent over $29 billion to educate about 170,000 medical students, basic science graduate students, and hospital residents. On the average, that is more than $170,000 apiece, per year. Of course, included in that figure are the salaries and stipends for the residents and graduate students. And medical schools do much else besides train physicians, including research and community service. But even taking those factors into account that per-student cost is quite high. And although tuition and fees account for only 4.1% of total medical school expenditures, it is not unusual for a student to graduate with $100,000 in debt accumulated for undergraduate and medical education.

NURSING[5]

Definition

Nursing has been defined by the American Nurses Association (ANA, 1990a, p. 8) as:

> Assessment, diagnosis, planning, intervention, and evaluation of human responses to health or illness; the provision of direct nursing care to individuals to restore optimum function, or to achieve a dignified death; . . . the provision of health counseling and education; the establishment of standards of practice for nursing care in all settings, including the development of nursing policies, procedures, and protocols for specific settings; . . . collaboration with other independently licensed health care professionals in case finding and the clinical management and execution of interventions and identified to be appropriate in a plan of care; and the administration of medication and treatments as prescribed by those persons qualified under the provision of the [law].

According to the Nursing Practice Act of New York State (Article 139, Para. 6902 of the State Education Law) (USNY [Nursing], 1995, p. 41):

> The practice of the profession of nursing as a registered professional nurse is defined as diagnosing and treating human responses to actual or potential health problems through such services as casefinding, health teaching, health counselling, and provision of care supportive to or restorative of life and well-being, and executing medical regimens prescribed by a licensed or otherwise legally authorized physician or dentist. A nursing regimen shall be consistent with and not vary any existing medical regimen.

Further the Act says (Para. 6901) (USNY [Nursing], 1995, p. 41):

> ''Diagnosing'' in the context of nursing practice means the identification of and discrimination between physical and psychosocial signs and symptoms essential to effective execution and management of the nursing regimen. Such diagnostic privilege is distinct from medical diagnosis. ''Treating'' means selection and performance of those therapeutic measures essential to the effective execution and management of the nursing regimen, and execution of any prescribed medical regimen. ''Human responses'' means

---

[5]For more detail on nursing, see chapter 5, ''Nursing,'' by Christine Kovner in *Jonas' health care delivery in the United States* (5th ed), Anthony Kovner (Ed.). New York: Springer Publishing Co., 1995.

> those signs, symptoms and processes which denote the individual's interaction with an actual or potential health problem.

According to the ANA (1995), the human responses with which nurses are concerned include: care and self-care processes; physiological and pathophysiological processes in areas ranging from rest and sleep to nutrition and sexuality; physical and emotional comfort, discomfort, and pain; emotional difficulties; decision and choice making; perceptual orientation; relationships and role performance; and social policies. Nurturing is the human characteristic basic to all nursing functions.

Some History

Women have provided the basic caring function in Western health care institutions since these institutions first appeared during the first millennium in Europe. The development of the modern nursing profession began in 1854 when Florence Nightingale traveled to the Russian Crimea in response to a British-government mandate to improve hospital care during the Crimean War. Her first problem was finding qualified nurses. Her second problem was to convince the military physicians that the care she and her nurses proposed to provide would not spoil the soldiers by "coddling the brutes." Third, she had to show that she had special skills and knowledge that could benefit the war effort.

Her nursing reforms eventually reduced hospital mortality from 60% to little more than 1%. This did not prevent repeated attempts to undermine the program and eliminate the nurses. In the United States Army, soldiers in the Spanish American War and World War I suffered while nurses struggled for the right to provide high-quality nursing care. It was not until 1944 that nurses in the military forces were granted temporary status as officers. Only in 1947 did Congress establish permanent Army and Navy Nurse Corps (Kalisch & Kalisch, 1978).

Categories of Nurses and Nursing Education

Nurses comprise the largest group of health professionals. As previously noted, in 1993 there were about 1,945,000 active registered nurses in the U.S. (*Health*, 1996, Table 101). Close to 1,200,000 of them had associate degrees or hospital-based nursing-school diplomas, more than 605,000 had baccalaureate degrees, and almost 160,000 had graduate degrees. The registered nurse:population ratio was about 755 per 100,000.

The heterogeneity of the U.S. health care system has created a need for nurses in many types of service. About half of all registered nurses work in hospitals. The balance work primarily in nursing homes for the chronically ill, public health agencies, schools, industrial clinics, nursing education, private medical or dental offices, and in private-duty positions.

There are three major groups of nurses: registered nurses (RNs), licensed practical nurses (LPNs), and nurses' aides (as well as orderlies, attendants, home health aides, and so on). RNs have the highest level of education, the most responsibility under the states' nurse practice acts, and the most authority. Generally, LPNs and aides function under the supervision of an RN.

"Registration" in nursing was originally a voluntary function of the nursing profession. It now means state licensure, at a significantly higher level of responsibility and authority than that accorded to the "licensed practical" nurse. To be a registered nurse one must have a high-school diploma and a diploma from a hospital-based program, or a bachelor of science in nursing (BSN) from a college or university, or, since 1952, an associate degree in nursing (ADN) from a 2-year college program. There are also master's and doctoral programs for registered nurses.

Licensed practical nurses, occasionally also called licensed vocational nurses (LVNs), may or may not have completed high school before entering a 12- to 18-month training program. LPN programs are operated by a variety of institutions including adult schools, junior colleges, and technical schools. Like RNs, LPNs must pass a state-supervised examination to become licensed, but their work requires a significantly lower level of skill and knowledge than does that of the RN. The education of the aides group is highly variable. Some study a formal educational program, for others the training is primarily on the job. In the work setting, the "mix" of RNs, LPNs, aides, orderlies, and so on is determined by the nature of patient care provided, government regulation, budget, and available manpower. Financial incentives have been provided in some state legislation to encourage facilities, such as nursing homes, to employ better qualified nursing staff.

Replacing Hospital Nurses

In the mid-1990s, some hospitals were attempting to replace RNs with technicians who would undergo very specific, focused, limited, short training programs. This could be seen as the offspring of a 1980s initiative by the American Medical Association. At that time, the AMA proposed the creation of the "registered care technician" (RCT) (Stein et al., 1990). The RCT would be trained in the hospital (like the original hospital-based diploma nurse) and primarily be responsible for carrying out the doctor's orders in such matters as medications, test-ordering, and discharge arrangements (like the original hospital-based diploma nurse). At about the same time the Center for Nursing of the American Hospital Association made a proposal for an occupation called the ''nurse extender'' (NE) (*American Hospital News*, 1990; Center for Nursing, 1989). The ANA commented that the AMA proposal ''was designed to return bedside nursing 'to a devalued, low paying, subservient field of practice' '' (Stein et al., 1990, p. 546).

Unlike the AMA's RCT, the AHA's NE would report to the nurse, not the doctor. The NE would be responsible for carrying out the many nursing tasks for which the RN education is not required (shades of the LPN). These included dealing with patient hygiene, nutritional and mobility needs, and clerical, supply-stocking, and patient-transport functions. However, among those tasks was *not* simply carrying out doctors' orders while bypassing the RN on the hospital floor.

With the managed-care-induced nurse surplus that had ensued by the mid-1990s (see below), neither of these proposals came to fruition as originally put forth. Some hospitals were experimenting on their own with a task-focused RCT-like worker to replace nurses at lower cost (Barter et al., 1992; Kunen, 1996; Lumsdon, 1995; Rosenthal, 1996), however, who would be trained within the hospital. It remains to be seen how successful (in several different senses of the word) that effort will be.

Nurses in Expanded Roles

Nurse practice has expanded since the days of Florence Nightingale. Each expansion first occurred through on-the-job experience and training. Only later would such preparation be formalized in an educational program. Thus, the first public-health nurses, who appeared during World War I, the first maternal and child health nurses, who came on the scene in the early 1920s, the first nurse anesthetists, nurse midwives, clinical nurse specialists, and nurse practitioners, were all prepared outside any formal educational system. In each instance, the initial informal efforts to create a new arena for nursing were followed by the establishment of standards, formal curricula in approved programs, and more recently, the preparation for advanced levels through master's-degree programs in universities.

Over time, the acceptance of new roles for nurses as first demonstrated in practice has led to continuing changes in nursing practice laws across the country. For example, in well-defined primary-care practice, an in-depth review of research carried out in the 1970s found no differences between the quality of care provided by qualified nurses and that provided by physicians (Record et al., 1981). Properly prepared nurses in advanced practice, the ''nurse practitioners,'' can provide much of primary ambulatory care, normal pregnancy care and delivery, and routine anesthesia at least as well as physicians.

In 1988, New York State, following the lead of a number of other states, formalized the nurse-practitioner role in its education law, to wit (USNY [Nursing] 1988, para. 6902 [3]):

> The practice of registered professional nursing by a nurse practitioner . . . may include the diagnosis of illness and physical conditions and the performance of therapeutic and corrective measures . . . in collaboration with a licensed physician . . . provided such services are performed in accordance with a written practice agreement and written practice protocols. The written practice agreement shall include explicit provisions for the resolution of any disagreement between the collaborating physician and the nurse practitioner regarding . . . diagnosis or treatment . . . within the scope of practice of both. To the extent the practice agreement does not so provide, then the collaborating physician's diagnosis or treatment shall prevail.

This sort of legislation opens the door for truly expanded nurse practice. That can be a boon to patients, especially in such areas as primary care.

From Nursing Shortage to Nursing Oversupply

Nursing shortages have appeared periodically in the United States (Aiken, 1982). One in the early 1950s led to the formalization of licensed practical nurse training and the requirements previously mentioned. As the 1990s began, another shortage was upon us (Aiken & Mullinix, 1987; ANA, 1990b; Secretary's Commission on Nursing, 1988). In 1990, the USDHHS estimated the nursing shortage to be about 200,000 (*Premier Focus*, 1990). It predicted shortages of about 350,000 in the year 2000, 520,000 in 2010, and 875,000 in 2020.

In 1988, the RN position-vacancy rate in hospitals was over 11%. In the face of this situation, nursing-school enrollments were actually declining and minority recruitment was lagging. Curiously, if half of the then approximately 400,000 RNs not working in nursing (ANA, 1990b) were to have done so, there would have been no nursing shortage.

At the time, authorities on the subject cited many reasons to account for the state of affairs (Igelhart, 1987). Among them were low salaries (the average starting salary for a staff nurse in 1988 was $25,000); limited chances for significant increases in pay over the life of a career (the average maximum salary for a *head* nurse in 1988 was $45,000); working conditions (high-tech work creates much stress, shift work is a serious problem); poor professional image; and widening career opportunities for women (both for those starting out in life and those who already are RNs). But the doctor–nurse relationship was considered key (Stein et al., 1990). As Aiken and Mullinix (1987, p. 645) pointed out: ''Much of the dissatisfaction of nurses with hospital practice is related to the absence of satisfying professional relationships with physicians.''

Among steps for which there was hope of implementation were (Helmer & McKnight, 1989): more creative solutions to the nights-and-weekends shifts problem, giving nurses more control over their own work, expanding nurse participation in hospital decision making, improving continuing professional education, restructuring the work of the nurse (part of which is the further extension of the nurse extender concept), developing better career ladders for nurses (although that would cost money).

At the center of it all, however, remained the need to further change the rules of the ''doctor–nurse game'' (Stein et al., 1990). After all, not all of those 400,000 RNs who in 1990 were not nursing chose to leave the profession simply because they were burned out, too old, having children, wanted to stay home, or thought some other line of work would be more fun.

But what a difference managed care made (Lumsdon, 1995). Hospitals began closing and shrinking in size. By the mid-1990s, not only was there no longer a nursing shortage, but nurse layoffs were occurring in certain areas of the country (Rosenthal, 1996). The University of California's Pew Center for the Health Professions (PHPC) predicted that 200,000 to 300,000 hospital-nurse positions could be eliminated by the year 2000. Regardless, however, as with physician supply no formal planning was occurring to deal in terms of supply, distribution, and role and function either with the existing nurse pool or nursing education.

THE PHYSICIAN ASSISTANT

The health profession of physician assistants (PA) has developed in the United States since the time of the Vietnam War (1965–1973).[6] The early development of the PA profession occurred just as the Vietnam War was

[6] At the 1972 Annual Meeting of the American Public Health Association there was a panel presentation on new health care delivery developments in Canada that included a discussion of the nurse practitioner. This author asked if there were P.A. programs in Canada. The speaker replied: ''We don't need to have P.A. programs. We have had no Vietnam War with the large number of returning medics to use and provide for. We need only nurse practitioner programs.''

getting underway. It received a big boost from the returning Vietnam veteran medical corpsmen. One can only speculate whether or not the PA profession would have been more than a blip on the radar screen of the history of health services had there been no war in Vietnam. Had the PA profession not proliferated, would the nurse-practitioner profession have become more prominent in the United States? But the war did occur, and whether or not the two are integrally related, the PA profession has become an established part of the U.S. health-services landscape. The PA profession has in fact become complex and multifaceted (Schafft & Cawley, 1987). The PA's role is to (Schafft & Cawley, 1987, p. 6):

- Approach a patient of any age group in any setting to elicit a detailed and accurate history, perform an appropriate physical examination, delineate problems, and record and present patient data.
- Analyze health status data obtained via interview, examination, and laboratory diagnostic studies and delineate health care problems in consultation with the physician.
- Formulate, implement, and monitor an individualized treatment and/or management plan for a patient in consultation with the physician.
- Instruct and counsel patients regarding compliance with the prescribed therapeutic regimen, normal growth and development, family planning, emotional problems of daily living, and health maintenance.
- Perform routine procedures essential to managing simple conditions produced by infection or trauma, assist in the management of more complex illness and injury, and initiate evaluations and therapeutic procedures in response to life-threatening situations.

It is estimated that a PA "can perform 80% of the routine functions of a primary care physician's practice," and "they are widely accepted by patients" (AAPA, 1996, p. 2).

From its beginnings the PA profession was conceived as an extension of the profession of medicine. It was not meant to be another separate profession like nursing. In each state, PA licensure is provided for under the medical practice act rather than under a separate law, as is the case with nursing. And although the gender balance within the PA profession has changed over the years to approximately 50:50 (AAPA, 1996), in the beginning it was predominately male. For these two reasons, many of the male chauvinist/power issues that cloud the relationship between physicians and nurses have not appeared.

In 1996 there were close to 80 PA training programs (AAPA, 1996). Most of them were situated in medical schools, teaching hospitals, or schools of the allied health professions in 4-year colleges. In 1996 there were about 26,000 PAs in the United States (AAPA, 1996). Although in the early days most PAs worked in primary care, by the 1980s specialization had become common.

In 1996, about half of the PA population worked in family practice (37.2% of the total), general internal medicine, general pediatrics, and obstetrics/gynecology, and another 22% were in surgery, close to 10% were in emergency medicine, with the balance in the other specialties. Some PAs work for individual physicians but most are employed in hospitals, clinics, group practices, and other organized health care settings. As do nurse practitioners, for the same kinds of patients PAs provide care that is comparable in quality to that provided by physicians.

HEALTH MANPOWER OUTSIDE THE HOSPITAL AND PHYSICIAN'S OFFICE

There are many settings in which health services are provided and many categories of health worker that provide them. In mental health centers, for example, the staff includes psychologists, psychiatric social workers and nurses, and carefully chosen support staff, in addition to psychiatrists. Community outreach workers are a new type of personnel trained in recent years by ambulatory care programs, both general and mental.

School health services are most often provided by a part-time or full-time school nurse, usually engaged by the local education authorities but sometimes assigned by the public health agency. School health physicians, who examine children to detect physical or mental disorders, are principally part-time private practitioners. In some large school districts, such as those of New York or Los Angeles, they may be employed full time. In some larger schools or schools districts, there may also be, for example, psychologists, social workers, audiologists, and dental hygienists.

In local health department centers public health nurses are the mainstay of the clinics that focus on preventive services, these nurses work with part-time physicians who are otherwise mainly in private practice. Other personnel in public health clinics include health educators, nutritionists or dietitians, sexually transmitted disease (STD) investigators, and various clerks. Beyond the personnel working in various clinics, public health agencies require sanitarians (to monitor environmental conditions), statisticians, community health educators with specialized skills, and sometimes persons trained specifically in family planning.

Turning to the pharmaceutical profession, in some countries pharmacies are devoted almost exclusively to the sale of medications. The number of pharmacists they produce is relatively smaller than in countries where the "drug store" also sells candy, tobacco products, and many other commodities. In the United States there are more than twice as many pharmacists per capita as there are in Great Britain, where the "chemist shop" dispenses only pharmaceutical drugs.

In sum, the health-personnel picture in the U.S. is a complex, expensive, and at times confusing one. On the technical side, it is highly developed, and many patients greatly benefit from the availability of so many different health care occupations with so much detailed education, training, and experience. There are both gaps and overlaps, however, and maldistribution is a significant problem. The introduction of comprehensive health planning would be a great help here, but as in all sectors of the U.S. health care delivery system, that development is a long way off (see chapter 7).

REFERENCES

AAPA (American Academy of Physician Assistants). *Information on the physician assistant profession.* Alexandria, VA: Author, May 1996.

Aiken L. H. (Ed.). *Nursing in the 1980's: Crises, opportunities, challenges.* Philadelphia: Lippincott, 1982.

Aiken, L. H., & Mullinix, C. F. The nurse shortage. *New England Journal of Medicine, 317,* 645, 1987.

American Hospital News. Hospitals' creative extender models help relieve nurse shortage. December 3, 1990.

AMA (American Medical Association). *Medical groups in the U.S.—A survey of practice characteristics (1996 ed.).* Chicago: Author, 1996.

ANA (American Nurses Association). *Suggested state legislation: Nursing Practice Act, Nursing Disciplinary Diversion Act, Prescriptive Authority Act.* Kansas City, MO: Author, 1990a.

ANA (American Nurses Association). Nursing shortage update. *Nurses,* Media Backgrounder: Author, February 1990b.

ANA (American Nurses Association). *Nursing's social policy statement.* Kansas City, MO: Author, 1995.

Barter, M., et al. Use of unlicensed assistive personnel by hospitals. *Nursing Economics, 12*(2), 82, 1994.

Barzansky, B., et al. Educational programs in US medical schools, 1995–96. *Journal of the American Medical Association, 276,* 714, 1996.

Bodenheimer, T., & Grumbach, K. Reimbursing physicians and hospitals. *Journal of the American Medical Association, 272,* 971, 1994.

Center for Nursing. *Restructuring the work load: Methods and models to address the nursing shortage.* Chicago: American Hospital Association, 1989.

Colwill, J. M. Education of the primary physician: A time for reconsideration? *Journal of the American Medical Association, 255,* 2643, 1986.

Donabedian, A., et al. *Medical care chartbook* (7th ed). Ann Arbor, MI: AUPHA Press, 1980.

Eisenberg, J. M. *Doctors' decisions and the cost of medical care.* Ann Arbor, MI: Health Administration Press, 1986.

Geyman, J. P. Training primary care physicians for the 21st century. *Journal of the American Medical Association, 255,* 2631, 1986.

Gillis, K. D., & Wilke, R. J. Employment patterns of physicians, 1983–1989. In M. L. Gonzalez & D. W. Emmons (Eds.), *Socioeconomic characteristics of medical practice, 1989.* Chicago: American Medical Association, 1989.

Helmer, F. T., & McKnight, P. Management strategies to minimize nursing turnover. *Health Care Management Review, 14*(1), 73, 1989.

Igelhart, J. K. Problems facing the nursing profession. *New England Journal of Medicine, 317,* 646, 1987.

IOM (Institute of Medicine). *The nation's physician workforce: Options for balancing supply and requirements.* Washington, DC: National Academy Press, 1996.

Kalisch, P. A., & Kalisch, B. J. *The advance of American nursing.* Boston: Little, Brown, 1978.

Krakower, J. Y., et al. Review of US medical school finances, 1994–95. *Journal of the American Medical Association, 276,* 720, 1996.

Kunen, J. The new hands-off nursing. *Time*, September 30, 1996.

Leape, L. L., et al. Relation between surgeons' practice volumes and geographic variation in the rate of carotid endarterectomy. *New England Journal of Medicine, 321,* 653, 1989.

Lumsdon, K. Faded glory. *Hospitals & Health Networks*, December 5, 1995, p. 31.

Mullan, F. Commentary on international medical graduates. *Public Health Reports, 110,* 667, 1995.

PHPC (Pew Health Professions Commission). *Critical challenges: Revitalizing the health professions for the twenty-first century.* San Francisco: UCSF Center for the Health Professions, Dec. 1995.

Premier Focus. Nursing. Westchester, IL: Premier Hospitals Alliance, October 1990.

Record, J., et al. *Primary care staffing in 1990: Physician replacement and cost savings.* New York: Springer Publishing Co., 1981.

Relman, A. S. The debate on primary-care manpower. *New England Journal of Medicine, 299,* 1305, 1978.

Rivo, M. L., et al. Managed health care: Implications for the physician workforce and medical education. *Journal of the American Medical Association, 274,* 712, 1995.

Rosenthal, E. Once in big demand, nurses are targets for hospital cuts. *New York Times*, August 19, 1996.

Ross, R. H., & Fineberg, H. V. *Innovations in physician education: The process and pattern of reform in North American medical schools*. New York: Springer Publishing Co., 1996.

Schafft, G. E., & Cawley, J. F. *The physician assistant*. Rockville, MD: Aspen Publishers, 1987.

Secretary's Commission on Nursing. *Final Report*. Washington, DC: USDHHS, December 1988.

Stein, L. I., et al. The doctor–nurse game revisited. *New England Journal of Medicine, 322,* 546, 1990.

USNY (University of the State of New York). *Medicine handbook*. Albany, NY: New York State Education Department, September 1995.

USNY (University of the State of New York). *Nursing handbook*. Albany, NY: New York State Education Department, 1988.

USNY (University of the State of New York). *Nursing handbook*. Albany, NY: New York State Education Department, May 1995.

Wachter, R. M., & Goldman, L. The emerging role of 'hospitalists' in the American health care system. *New England Journal of Medicine, 335,* 514, 1996.

Wennberg, J. E. Dealing with medical practice variations: A proposal for action. *Health Affairs, 3,* 6, 1984.

Wennberg, J. E. *The Dartmouth atlas of health care*. Chicago: American Hospital Association, 1996.

White, K. L. Organization and delivery of personal health services—Public policy issues. *Milbank Memorial Fund Quarterly*, January, 1968. Reprinted in J. B. McKinlay (Ed.), *Politics and Law in Health Care Policy*, New York: Prodist, 1973.

Chapter **3**

Institutions: Hospitals

SOME HISTORY

Historically, for the provision of personal health care the hospital has been the institutional center of the health care delivery system (Knowles, 1980). In its "teaching" incarnation the modern hospital is also the center of much undergraduate and graduate clinical training for many health professions, and continuing health sciences education, both formal and informal. In addition, some teaching hospitals are major medical research institutions.

Traditionally, the hospital has been an important workplace for most U.S. physicians (in addition to their private offices), and the only place where they are likely to be subject to peer review of their professional work. With the advent of managed care, both of these features are changing (see below and chapter 8).

While just before the turn of the 20th century a person entering a hospital had less than a 50% chance of leaving it alive, today most patients can expect to benefit from a hospital stay (Rosenberg, 1979). About 97% of patients admitted leave the hospital alive, sitting or walking. The hospital has evolved from a place where a person went to spare his family the anguish of watching him die, to a multiservice institution providing interdisciplinary medical care to ambulatory as well as bed patients.

The word "hospital" shares its Latin root with the words "hostel" and "hotel." Most frequently under church sponsorship, the institution originated in the Middle Ages as a place of refuge for the poor, the sick, and the just plain weary. In modern times hospitals provide in- and outpatient diagnostic and treatment services for the poor with short- and long-term health problems (Freymann, 1974; Stern, 1946), and for the acutely ill of all social classes (Freymann, 1974).

In the European settlements in America, the earliest hospitals were infirmaries attached to poorhouses. (A poorhouse was an institution operated by a local government authority to house persons who were: unemployed; orphaned or abandoned children; the ill elderly and/or those otherwise incapable of self-care; and the mentally ill/retarded.) The first of these was established at Henricopolis in Virginia (1612), the next not until 1732 in Philadelphia (Stern, 1946).

The first public institution designed solely for the care of the sick was the "pesthouse" built in 1794 on Manhattan Island north of what was then New York City at a place called Belle Vue ("beautiful vista"). In a reverse of the earlier pattern, the New York City public workhouse (a variation of the poorhouse) was moved to the grounds of the "pesthouse" in 1816. The famous Bellevue Hospital is still at that location. *Non*government charity (private "voluntary") hospitals to care for the poor were also established in the American colonies during the 18th century (Freymann, 1974). The first of these was the Pennsylvania Hospital in Philadelphia, founded by Benjamin Franklin in 1751.

By 1873 there were an estimated 178 hospitals in the United States. Many of them happened to be solely for the mentally ill, however (Stevens, 1971). At about that time the development of modern medical science was underway, and a general hospital-building boom began. By the early 20th century a patient admitted to a general hospital had a better than even chance of getting out alive. That milestone was achieved largely through the development of general hospital hygiene, asepsis, and surgical anesthesia. After the turn of the century, medical care quickly became far too complex for the physician to be able to carry his entire armamentarium in his black bag. By 1910 general hospitals had been established in many communities. There were nearly 4,400 of them, with a total of 421,000 beds (Stevens, 1971). It was the continued rapid advance of medical science that led to the continued expansion of the hospital system and of individual hospitals, and the evolution of hospitals as the center of the medical care system (MacEachern, 1962).

BASIC DATA

Sources

The American Hospital Association (AHA) is the primary agency that counts and classifies hospitals in the United States. For the hospital world it regularly publishes *The AHA Guide to the Health Care Field* (AHA [*Guide*], 1995) and its companion, *Hospital Statistics* (AHA [*Stats.*], 1995). The former lists each AHA registered hospital, giving its basic characteristics, as well as other valuable information (see Appendix II).

The latter presents summary statistical data about U.S. hospitals. A few selected summaries of AHA and other hospital statistical data are published in *Health: United States* (see chapter 1). This chapter uses AHA definitions and data, except as otherwise noted.

Primary Definitions

Hospital size. This is determined by the number of beds: the average number of beds, cribs, and pediatric bassinets regularly maintained (set up and staffed for use) for inpatients during the reporting period (AHA [*Stats.*], 1995).

Hospital type. There are nine types of hospitals: community (see below), federal, long-term, hospital units of institutions (such as prisons and universities), psychiatric, those specifically for tuberculosis and other respiratory diseases, chronic disease, mental retardation, and alcoholism and other chemical dependencies.

The AHA's all-inclusive descriptor for the majority of hospitals, the "community hospital" (Igelhart, 1993, p. 372) is defined as "all nonfederal short term general or other special hospitals, whose facilities are available to the [general] public." The "other special hospital" category includes: obstetrics and gynecology; eye, ear, nose, and throat; rehabilitation; orthopedic; and other individually described specialty services. The term "general hospital" includes all short-term hospitals other than the named special hospitals and those in the "other special" category, regardless of ownership (AHA [*Stats.*], 1995).

Mode of ownership. There are two principal types of ownership: private and public. In turn, there are two categories of private hospital, differentiated by the mode of distribution of surplus income: "investor owned" for profit (formerly called "proprietary"), and not for profit (voluntary). There are also two categories of public hospital: federal and nonfederal (that is, state and local).

Length of patient stay. There are two categories defined by length of stay: "long term" and "short term," respectively 30 days or more and fewer than 30 days.

The division among hospitals by type noted above was established some time ago, as described by Freymann (1974, p. 47):

> The mold from which today's health care system was cast took its shape around 1850. There were still relatively few general hospitals or health facilities of any type in Britain [our most important medical *organizational* forebear] and the fledgling United States, but the institutional organization of health care was already firmly established. Separate administration and

staffing of the curative services for acute, chronic, and psychiatric illnesses became such a strong precedent that it continues even when all three components have a common source of support, as they do now in Britain.

Some Numbers

Overall

In the first instance a hospital is described by size, type, ownership mode, whether it is short term or long term (defined by length of patient stay), by the average daily census (the average number of beds occupied on a given day, other than by newborns, usually computed on an annual basis), and occupancy rate (the average proportion of total beds occupied). Table 3.1 presents data for the major classes of hospital for 1994. Most common is the voluntary general short-term hospital, followed in number by the local government general short-term hospital. The other major groups are the federal short-term hospitals, the state mental hospitals, and the proprietary short-term hospitals.

TABLE 3.1 Major Hospital Groups, United States, Basic Characteristics, 1994

Class	Federal	Nonfederal psychiatric	Not-for-profit community	For-profit community	State and local community
Characteristic					
Hospitals	307	691	3139	719	1371
Beds (thousands)	84	121	637	101	164
Annual admissions (thousands)	1588	749	22704	3035	4979
Average daily census (thousands)	63	97	413	50	104
Occupancy (%)	75	80	65	50	63
Average length of stay (days)	NA	NA	6.6	6.1	7.6

Source: AHA (*Stats.*), 1995, Table 3A.

As of 1994, there were about 1.1 million beds in a total of about 6,375 hospitals, with an average daily census of about 745,000 patients, and an overall occupancy rate of about 66% (AHA [*Stats.*], 1995). The hospital profile has changed over time. In 1978, a peak year, when the U.S. population was close to 40,000,000 fewer than it was in 1994, there were almost 1.4 million beds in 7,015 hospitals of all kinds, with an average daily census of 1.04 million patients, and an overall occupancy rate of 75.5% (AHA, 1979). As of 1990, there were about 1.2 million beds in a total of about 6,700 hospitals, with an average daily census about 850,000 patients, and an overall occupancy rate of about 70% (AHA, 1990).

In 1994, there were about 5,200 community hospitals, with 902,000 beds, close to 31 million admissions, and an average daily census of 568,000. The peak number of community hospitals in the United States, 5,881, was reached in 1977. Between 1964 and 1978 the number of community-hospital beds increased from 721,000 to 975,000, or 35%. During the same period, reflecting the decline in the number of small hospitals, the average number of beds per hospital increased by 32% (AHA, 1979).

Teaching Hospitals

In the past the AHA has used the term "teaching hospital" to refer to hospitals providing undergraduate and/or graduate teaching for medical students and/or medical house staff (interns, residents, and specialty fellows) (see also chapter 2). The term was not applied to hospitals with teaching programs for other health care providers. Although the AHA formerly presented data for the teaching hospitals separately, that data is now subsumed under the by-type categories of which the teaching hospitals are a part.

In one of the last years for which teaching-hospital data were presented separately, 1989, there were 1,054 teaching community hospitals (about 19% of all community hospitals) with 393,000 beds (more than 42% of all beds in community hospitals) (AHA, 1990). Their average size was about 370 beds, whereas the average size for all community hospitals was about 170 beds. They provided over 14 million admissions (almost 46% of the total to community hospitals), and, on the average day, cared for over 47% of all community-hospital patients. They provided almost one half of all visits to community-hospital outpatient departments. Their occupancy rate was 74.6% and the average length of stay was 7.5 days. In terms of both professional education and service, teaching hospitals have an importance in the hospital system quite out of proportion to their number.

Distribution and Relative Bed Supply

In 1948, there were approximately 3.4 nonfederal general medical and surgical hospital beds per 1,000 civilian resident population (AHA, 1990; U.S. Bureau of the Census, 1990). By 1976, the community hospital bed:population ratio was 4.5 beds per 1,000. By 1989, the ratio had declined to 3.85, and by 1994 it had reached 3.46, about where it was in 1948. Primarily because of a post-World War II hospital construction program known as ''Hill–Burton'' (after its two original Congressional sponsors), however, the geographical distribution of beds was quite different in 1994 than it had been in 1948.

Under Hill–Burton, many rural hospitals were built in areas that previously had had no direct access to modern health services. Improvements in bed distribution and increases in bed supply since World War II, which provided access for many persons for whom hospital services were formerly unavailable, have been regarded as an outstanding national achievement. It turns out that without a comprehensive health-care-planning system in place, however, the hospital industry rather overshot the mark, creating many hospitals, particularly in the West and South, that now have low occupancy rates and many permanently empty beds. A good deal of money was wasted in the process.

Hospital closure secondary to overbedding is the reason why in recent years the national bed/population ratio has been declining, although again haphazardly, without a plan. Under the pressure of managed care and ''free market'' competition the hospital bed supply should continue to shrink for some years to come. In the continued absence of any rational or national health care planning system, the possible outcomes this time around are all too predictable.

In theory, the number of beds needed for a given geographic region is a function of the number of patient days of hospital care medically required by the population (expressed as a projected average daily census) and the working occupancy level deemed appropriate for the hospitals of a given area (Sattler & Bennett, 1975), usually 90%–95%. As noted, however, in certain sections of the country, hospital beds have not always been built in accordance with such a rational formula.

Other factors that led to hospital construction include: demands by the local physicians for facilities for their use, local wealth and other available sources of funds, civic pride, and competition with other institutions. Much as it may come as a shock to some readers, in the health care arena the thought, ''Well, if the hospital down the road has an ultraoxymegatron, then, you know, we've got to have one too'' has been known to obtain from time to time.

In the past, once built, the availability of a hospital bed promoted its use (Klarman, 1965). This phenomenon, "a built bed is a filled bed," was popularly termed "Roemer's Law" (Roemer, 1961). But not all patients required hospitalization on medical grounds. Among the nonmedical reasons for hospital admission were patient and physician convenience, physician and hospital pecuniary gain, and the availability of hospital-payment insurance. With various regulatory controls placed on hospital admissions since the mid-1970s, however, the occupancy rates did decline, as noted previously. Managed care utilization controls (see chapter 8) are further reducing hospital occupancy rates.

Unfilled beds happen to be costly to maintain. Many hospital costs are either fixed or they can be varied in the face of short-term changes in utilization only with difficulty. These costs include those for capital construction and equipment, mortgage and bond interest payments, and personnel and utility costs. Only expenditures for food and consumable supplies do not have to be made when a bed is empty in a hospital unit that is open. For these reasons, it has been estimated that on a short-term basis an empty bed costs about 70% as much to maintain as does a filled one (Blue Cross/Blue Shield). The only way to really save money in the hospital sector is to close beds and eliminate those high fixed costs.

Characteristics of Hospitalized Patients

Considerable data on the characteristics of hospitalized patients are available from the National Hospital Discharge Survey produced annually by the National Center for Health Statistics (Graves & Gillum, 1996) of the USDHHS. In 1994, excluding newborns, there were about 30.8 million discharges from nonfederal short-stay hospitals. The average length of stay was 5.7 days. Persons 65 and over accounted for 37% of all discharges. Half of all discharges had a diagnosis in one of just four diagnostic groups: diseases of the circulatory system, the respiratory system, and the digestive system, and "supplementary classifications" (including deliveries of newborns).

There were more than a million discharges in each of five specific diagnostic categories: heart disease (4.1 million), obstetrical deliveries (3.9 million), cancer (1.4 million), psychoses (1.2 million), and pneumonia (1.2 million). Close to 41 million diagnostic and therapeutic procedures were performed, almost 75% of them in four diagnostic groups: "miscellaneous," obstetrical procedures, operations on the digestive system and operations on the cardiovascular system.

HOSPITAL STRUCTURE

Introduction

Hospitals have a complex structure and a variety of administrative operating divisions. Traditionally the principal ones are: medical (the physicians), nursing, other diagnostic and therapeutic support, financial, personnel, hotel, and community relations. Most hospitals provide services both to inpatients placed in a bed and to outpatients (see chapter 4) who come to an emergency department, an outpatient clinic, or for a diagnostic or therapeutic service (such as an ambulatory surgery unit) for a procedure not requiring hospitalization.

Hospital Administration

Hospital administration keeps the institution up and running in all areas other than direct patient care. Its major responsibilities include: finance, personnel, community/public relations, and the "hotel" services: maintenance, housekeeping, laundry, and dietary (cooking and delivery of meals).

A popular buzzword of the mid-1990s in hospital management was "reengineering." The process it describes often has nothing to do with engineering per se. Rather, it is jargon for what used to be called the planning-and-development process applied to program redesign. It usually focuses on the integration of traditionally separate hospital functions that produce patient events such as admission, inpatient management, and discharge planning (Bischoff, 1996).

Reengineering attempts to achieve "extensive, radical" changes in hospital operations by designing programs the staffing, administration, and operation of which cross traditional departmental or unit lines. In theory, the process discards basic, preexisting assumptions and starts from the ground up. This does not always happen, however. And so, in some of those hospitals that have tried reengineering and the many that have not, administration is still organized around divisions. It is to a consideration of some of them that we shall next turn.

Medical Division

The Departments

The medical division is organized along the lines of the several medical specialties. There is no universal logic to the categorization, however, and there are certain crossovers and overlaps, as the reader will note.

Some are defined by the class of procedure used, some by the age or gender of their primary patient-population group, and some by the organ or organ system that is their purview.

The major medical departments are as follows:

- *Internal medicine*: diagnosis and therapy for adults, involving one or more internal organs or the skin, not requiring physical alteration of the body.
- *Surgery*: diagnosis and therapy in which physical alteration of the patient's body is usually the focus of the physician's intervention.
- *Pediatrics*: diagnosis and therapy for children, primarily using non-surgical techniques.
- *Obstetrics/gynecology*: diagnosis and therapy focusing on the female sexual/reproductive system using both surgical and nonsurgical interventions.
- *Psychiatry*: diagnosis and therapy for people of all ages with psychological and emotional problems, using counselling, pharmaceutical, and other interventions.

Other medical departments organized around organs and organ systems in which the physicians use both surgical and nonsurgical interventions include: ophthalmology (eye); otolaryngology (ear, nose, and throat); urology (male sexual/reproductive system, and the renal system for both males and females); orthopedics (bones and joints); neurology (nonsurgical) and neurosurgery (both concerned with the nervous system), and so on.

Radiology, the use of X-ray and other radiation sources, is a medical department with a primarily diagnostic function, although radiotherapy is also an important of radiology's function. In recent years, several non-X-ray internal diagnostic techniques, such as computerized axial tomography (CAT) scanning and magnetic resonance imaging (MRI) have been developed. They are usually within the purview of the department of radiology (in some institutions now called "Diagnostic Imaging" to reflect the new technology). In some hospitals radiotherapy (also called therapeutic nuclear medicine) has been separated from diagnostic radiology and its newer cousins.

In medical practice pathology serves only a diagnostic function, both before and after treatment. Traditionally, anesthesiology has been principally concerned with preparing patients to be surgically operated on without pain or discomfort during the procedure. More recently, some anesthesiologists are participating in emergent or "critical care" medicine, whereas others have expanded their practice to include general "pain management."

Medical Staff Organization

The physician is traditionally described both as a guest in the hospital and as its primary customer. The hospital has been sometimes described as the doctors' workshop. Except when a physician chooses to run a hospital for profit, however, he has no personal responsibility to see that the hospital is available to provide care for his patients. Nor does she carry any financial liability for the success or failure of the hospital, unless, again, she is an owner.

A physician is largely free to order whatever tests or treatments deemed necessary for the patient. Thus the physician is a major determinant of hospital costs, even though traditionally he has born no personal responsibility for them. The physician also influences the growth and expansion of the institution. Physician behavior is thus a major factor in the continuing rise in health care costs.

Under managed care, in certain institutions, these relationships are changing. For example, in an arrangement called the ''physician–hospital organization'' (PHO), groups of medical staff are joining with hospital corporations to negotiate contracts with third-party payers, often a managed care organization (MCO, most often an HMO, see chapter 8) to provide both medical and hospital services (Kongstvedt & Plocher, 1996). Assuming that the payments from the MCO to the PHO are made on an other than fee-for-service basis, and increasingly they are (Hudson, 1996), such an arrangement does put the medical staff at some financial risk should patient utilization exceed projections.

In the traditional hospital–medical staff arrangement, in exchange for the privilege of admitting patients, the physician participates in the self-governance of the medical staff and may have to share the load for providing care in areas of the hospital for which the medical staff accepts collective responsibility, such as the emergency room or outpatient clinic. A wide variety of medical staff patterns of organization exist. Roemer and Friedman's (1971) review is still valid.

There are many medical staff committees responsible for overseeing the physicians' work. They include: the executive committee, which provides overall coordination and sets general policy; the joint conference committee, which serves as liaison between the medical staff and the hospital's governing board; the credentials committee, which reviews applications to join the medical staff and controls the periodic reappointment process; the infections control committee, which is responsible for preventing infections and monitoring and correcting any outbreaks that do occur; the pharmacy and therapeutics committee, which reviews pharmacologic agents for inclusion in the list of drugs approved for use in the hospital.

There are also the tissue committee, which reviews all surgical procedures that produce ''bodily tissues;'' the medical records committee, which is responsible for certifying the completeness and clinical accuracy of the documentation of patient care; and finally, the quality-assurance committee, which undertakes the responsibilities that its name implies.

Other Health Care Divisions

The other principal health care division is nursing (see chapter 2). The nonphysician diagnostic-and-therapeutic services, which may or may not be administratively attached to one of the medical departments, include: laboratory (usually under the direction of the department of pathology); electrocardiography (usually a part of internal medicine); electroencephalography (part of neurology); radiotherapy technology (diagnostic imaging); pharmacy; clinical psychology; social service; inhalation therapy (often part of anesthesiology or pulmonary medicine); nutrition as therapy; physical, occupational, and speech therapy (often attached to the department of rehabilitation medicine, if there is one); home care; and medical records (AHA, 1990).

Hospital Governance in the Private Sector

The typical not-for-profit hospital has a self-perpetuating Board of Trustees. Usually prominent in its membership are persons who give or raise substantial sums of money for the hospital or represent important community institutions such as major employers and banks. The person carrying the title of ''President'' of the hospital is either the leader of the Board of Trustees, or the paid Chief Executive Officer of the hospital. In the former case, the top paid person is usually called the Executive Director or Executive Vice-President. In the latter case the Board is headed by a chairman. In theory, the Board of Directors sets policy and the Chief Executive Officer carries it out. In practice, the situation is often as complex as it is in any medium- to large-size modern corporation.

For-profit hospitals may have a governance structure similar to that of the voluntaries, with Board seats held by the owners or their representatives, or they may be run directly by the owner(s). All hospitals operate under the license and supervision (closer in some states than in others) of an agency of state government.

PUBLIC GENERAL HOSPITALS

The public *general* hospital (recall that there are other classes such as veterans [see chapter 6] and mental) was defined by the Commission on Public-General Hospitals of the American Hospital Association (1978, p.

v) as ''short term general and certain special hospitals excluding Federal (those operated by the Department of Defense and the Department of Veterans Affairs), psychiatric, and tuberculosis hospitals, that are owned by state and local governments.''

The public hospital sector is shrinking along with the hospital sector in general. In 1981, at the beginning of the Reagan presidency, there were 1,772 state and local general hospitals. As of 1989, there were 1,390 local government and 92 state government general hospitals with a total of about 170,000 beds (AHA, 1990). By 1994, there were a total of 1,371 state and local government community hospitals with a total of about 164,000 beds, and an occupancy rate of 63%.

Public general hospitals provide care for many persons unable to get care elsewhere: the poor, the homeless, the street prostitute, the destitute drug addict or alcoholic, the disruptive poor psychiatric patient, the low-income elderly, and the prisoner. In certain areas, they are the only source of care for the patients with special medical problems: the badly burned, the at-risk newborn, the high-risk mother, and the victim of criminal or noncriminal life-threatening trauma. Although only a minority of hospitals are under public ownership, in a nation without universal health care cost coverage, they play a role of importance beyond their numbers, while at the same time their numbers are declining (Verghese, 1996).

THE HOSPITAL IN THE PRESENT ERA

Problems

First, hospitals have been costly to build and maintain. And they still are, even as their numbers shrink and the pace of new construction/renovation slows markedly. Second, there is an imbalance in the hospital sector between acute, long-term, and ambulatory care. The high costs of inpatient hospital care are exacerbated by the inadequate supply of affordable, long-term care beds for patients who have recovered from the acute phase of their illness but still need high-quality care in bed.

Beyond that, as noted by Rogatz (1980) there is a pressing need for appropriate housing with social and support services for the elderly who cannot live entirely on their own in ordinary housing, but nevertheless do not need institutionalization of any kind. If anything, this situation has gotten worse in the intervening years.

The third major problem concerns the mode by which most physicians taking care of patients in hospitals have traditionally been paid, and the influence that physicians have over hospital operations. As noted previously, the physician has traditionally made most of the decisions on the commitment and use of hospital resources. Yet it usually has been the patient or his insurer who pay the doctor. Thus, the physician has neither a direct financial relationship to the hospital, nor any responsibility for its financial health.

A comparable situation would be if modern schoolboards were to provide everything necessary for education except payment of the teachers, who would proceed to collect fees directly from the students. Indeed this is the way teachers were paid before the educational reforms of the mid-19th century. As noted, managed care is beginning to change some of these relationships in some hospitals in some areas of the country.

Fourth, hospitals have internal problems with vertically organized administrative structures that are not well integrated at the service levels. In many hospitals the vertical lines of authority of the medical staff, nursing, and support/hotel services meet only in the office of the director. In some cases, however, they never meet. This kind of separation can make it very difficult to provide integrated patient-care programs in which those at the functional level follow in one direction in order to best meet patient needs (Jonas, 1973).

A fifth problem is the programmatic and sometimes philosophical isolation of many hospitals from the real health and medical problems of their communities. This does not apply solely to short-term general hospitals. For example, in many hospitals outpatient services have had a distinctly second-class status, preventive medicine is practiced to a minimal extent (although that situation is improving), home care and rehabilitation services have been treated as luxuries, community-based chronic disease control programs are not undertaken, and mental hospitals have little to do with community mental health. Although change is surely occurring, some hospitals have resolutely turned inward, wishing that everyone would just go away and leave them to do their job as they see it: taking care of sick people in bed.

Sixth, as should be apparent from what has already been said in this chapter, hospitals have been plunged into the era of managed care without a good deal of warning or preparation and certainly no formal planning, whether at the state or national level. A major thrust of managed care has been to reduce hospital usage. As noted, hospitals, mainly smaller ones, have been closing, and some larger ones have closed some bed units, leading to the reduction in hospital numbers and bed supply already noted.

These developments have led to, among other things, a flurry of hospital mergers and takeovers, as well as the formation of an ever-increasing number of "hospital networks." The latter is some kind of formal relationship among a group of hospitals, usually with a major tertiary-care teaching hospital at its center.

Certain economies of scale and divisions of labor can be achieved with such arrangements. Consider the climate of the mid-1990s, however: no national health care program, an increasing number of uninsured and underinsured persons (Weissman, 1996), and managed care organizations simply looking for the best deal in making their contracts with hospitals to provide services for the MCO's beneficiaries. If hospitals, especially expensive teaching hospitals, simply are looking to a network as the means for keeping their beds filled and do not contemplate further major *service* reorganization that will deemphasize expensive inpatient care and enable them to close expensive beds, some of them will not be able to stay afloat in the current era.

Solutions

Complex problems do not have simple solutions, and there are no panaceas. But in the context of a program of universal financial entitlement to health services, a variety of approaches to hospital reform are available. For one example, we can turn once again to Freymann (1974), who developed the "mission-oriented hospital" concept.

The mission-oriented hospital has two principal attributes: (1) each hospital has a mission defined and continuously modified by the specific needs of the community it serves, and (2) the rational planning process provides individuality and flexibility (Freymann, 1974). Freymann recognized that (1974, p. 247):

> The word "hospital" itself presents a problem, for today it connotes a building that houses patients. I think "hospital" could be used in a different sense to signify a dynamic complex of facilities and skilled personnel organized to provide all types of health services.

The mission-oriented approach would make the hospital into a health center rather than an illness center, ending what Freymann (1974) called the "tyranny of the bed." The hospital would respond to the needs of its community in a rational, planned, dynamic manner. By definition, the acute/chronic/preventive distinctions would become relics of the past.

The present-day administrative problems would not be resolved automatically by a mission-oriented approach. Rather, they would *have* to be solved in order to accomplish mission orientation. This approach demands an administrative structure that is functionally decentralized to operate integrated programs requiring staff teams at the patient-care level, not one that has vertically organized reporting lines separating health care providers into independent hierarchies.

This outcome might be achieved through managed-care induced hospital reorganizations, especially networking and the development of integrated delivery systems (Kongstvedt & Plocher, 1996). However, because mission orientation as defined by Freymann requires, at least in part, a focus on issues other than the shape of the bottom line, achieving that outcome might be beyond the capabilities of managed care as it is presently structured. Furthermore, it is highly unlikely that mission orientation can be achieved in the absence of a national health care program (see chapter 9).

Another approach that is receiving quite a bit of attention in the 1990s is the "hospital-within-a-hospital" administrative structure, designed to provide "patient-focused care" (*Medical Staff News*, 1996). The former "reorganizes the hospital's activities, resources, and personnel around the hospital's strategic business units by bringing together related clinical product lines" (*Medical Staff News*, 1996, p. 1). They are organized, for example, around the following patient care units: medical, surgical, cardiovascular, maternal/child, and mental health.

The traditional tripartite vertical structure in the hospital, medical services, nursing services, and administrative/support services is thus replaced by a collaborative management team for each designated patient-care unit. The idea is to integrate the medical, nursing, and administrative functions at the patient-service level, with shared management responsibility and authority for all aspects of operations.

Patient-focused care itself is defined as: "A method of changing the processes and systems involved with delivering care to patients within each patient care unit" (*Medical Staff News*, 1996, p. 1). It remains to be seen whether this kind of reorganization is merely a change of labels on the jar without changing what is inside, or whether it achieves some significant changes in how the hospital operates and delivers patient care.

Long-Term Care: The Example of Nursing Homes[1]

"Long-term care is a range of health, personal care, social, and housing services provided to people who have lost or have never developed the capacity to care for themselves independently as a result of chronic illness or mental or physical disability" (Richardson, 1995, p. 194). There is a

[1]Long-term care deserves a much more complete discussion than we have room for in this book. Much of this short section is based on "Long Term Care" by Hila Richardson, chapter 8 in *Jonas' health care delivery in the United States* (5th ed.), A. Kovner (Ed.), New York: Springer Publishing Co., 1995. The reader is referred to this excellent chapter for more detail on nursing homes in particular and long-term care in general.

group of long-term care institutions other than long-term hospitals, which are generically called "nursing homes." Their number has increased significantly since the 1930s, although it is declining in the present era.

Formerly classified according to the level of skill involved in the care they gave, beginning in 1990 all nursing homes eligible to receive federal third-party reimbursement for the care they provide are called nursing facilities. In 1986 there were over 16,000 such institutions of 25 beds or more, with over 1,600,000 beds (NCHS, 1990). Occupancy rates averaged over 90%, and there were over 540 beds per 1,000 persons aged 85 or older. By 1991 there were under 15,000 nursing homes with about 1.5 million beds, providing just under 500 beds per 1,000 persons 85 years of age or older (NCHS, 1996).

About 75% of nursing homes are under for-profit ownership, with 20% in the voluntary sector, and 5% owned by government agencies (Richardson, 1995). Fewer than 70% of the beds are found in the proprietary units. More than half of the financial support for nursing homes comes from public funds, much of it Medicaid, as Medicare provides little long-term-care coverage. In fact, in the mid-1990s, although two thirds of persons covered by Medicaid were welfare recipients, two thirds of Medicaid expenditures went to pay for nursing home care, not all of it for people who were in the low-income group for the whole of their lives.

Chronic problems with the quality of long-term care provoke periodic exposés and outcries for reform. But because any institutional care is expensive, the long-term solution to the long-term care problem probably lies with improved home-care services and improved health promotive, disease preventive self-care programs for the rapidly increasing number of elderly persons in the United States.

REFERENCES

AHA (American Hospital Association). *The AHA guide to the health care field, 95/6*. Chicago: Author, 1995.

AHA (American Hospital Association). *Hospital statistics, 1979*. Chicago: Author, 1979.

AHA (American Hospital Association). *Hospital statistics 1990–91*. Chicago: Author, 1990.

AHA (American Hospital Association). *Hospital statistics 95/6*. Chicago: Author, 1995.

Bischoff, T. Notes. Course in academic health center administration, Wagner School. New York University, April 9, 1996.

Commission on Public-General Hospitals. *The future of the public-general hospital.* Chicago: Hospital Research and Educational Trust, 1978.

Freymann, J. G. *The American health care system: Its genesis and trajectory.* New York: Medcom Press, 1974.

Graves, E. J., & Gillum, B. S. 1994 summary: National Hospital Discharge Survey. *Advance Data*, No. 278, October 3, 1996.

Hudson, T. What PHOs know. *Hospitals and Health Networks*, Sept. 5, 1996, p. 54.

Igelhart, J. K. The American health care system: Community hospitals. *New England Journal of Medicine, 329,* 372, 1993.

Jonas, S. Some thoughts on primary care: Problems in implementation. *International Journal of Health Services, 3,* 177, 1973.

Klarman, H. E. *The economics of health.* New York: Columbia University Press, 1965.

Knowles, J. The hospital. In S. J. Williams (Ed.), *Issues in health services.* New York: Wiley, 1980, Chapter 8.

Kongstvedt, P. R., & Plocher, D. W. Integrated health care delivery systems. In P. R. Kongstvedt (Ed.), *The managed health care handbook*, Gaithersburg, MD: Aspen, 1996.

MacEachern, M. T. *Hospital organization and management.* Berwyn, IL: Physician's Record Co., 1962.

Medical Staff News (University Hospital at Stony Brook, NY). Hospital-within-a-hospital takes shape. *Medical Staff News, 1*(2), 1, 1996.

NCHS (National Center for Health Statistics). *Health United States, 1989.* Hyattsville, MD: DHHS Pub. No. (PHS) 90-1232, 1990.

NCHS (National Center for Health Statistics). *Health United States, 1995.* Hyattsville, MD: DHHS Pub. No. (PHS) 96-1232, 1996.

Richardson, H. Long term care. In A. Kovner (Ed.), *Jonas' Health Care Delivery in the United States* (5th ed.). New York: Springer Publishing Co., 1995.

Roemer, M. Bed supply and hospital utilization: A natural experiment. *Hospitals, J.A.H.A.*, November 1961.

Roemer, M. I., & Friedman, J. W. *Doctors in hospitals.* Baltimore, MD: Johns Hopkins Press, 1971.

Rogatz, P. M. Directions of health system for the new decade. *Hospitals*, January 1, 1980, p. 67.

Rosenberg, C. E. The origins of the American hospital system. *Bulletin of the New York Academy of Medicine, 55,* 10, 1979.

Sattler, F. L., & Bennett, M. D. *A statistical profile of short-term hospitals in the United States as of 1973.* Minneapolis, MN: Interstudy, 1975.

Stern, B. J. *Medical services by government.* New York: Commonwealth Fund, 1946.

Stevens, R. *American medicine and the public interest.* New Haven, CT: Yale University Press, 1971.

U.S. Bureau of the Census. *Statistical abstract of the United States, 1990.* Washington, DC: U.S.G.P.O. 1979.

Verghese, A. My hospital, dying a slow death. *New York Times*, November 30, 1996.

Weissman, J. Uncompensated hospital care. *Journal of the American Medical Association, 276*, 823, 1996.

Chapter 4

Institutions: Primary and Ambulatory Care

PRIMARY CARE

Introduction

Primary care and ambulatory care go together like apple pie and ice cream. This is so even though not all primary care is delivered in an ambulatory setting, nor is all ambulatory care primary care. Nevertheless, as they are in most instances so closely associated, they are covered in the same chapter.

As noted in chapter 1, by sheer volume primary health care services are primary. But primary care has proved difficult to define precisely. In 1977 the Institute of Medicine reviewed 33 different definitions of the term (Ruby, 1977). More recently, Dr. Barbara Starfield (1992, p. 1365) has provided one normative definition, covering both what primary *is* and in the best of all possible worlds what it *ought* to be:

> Primary care is the means by which the two goals of a health services system—optimization of health and equity in distributing resources—are balanced. It is the basic level of care provided equally to everyone. It addresses the most common problems in the community by providing preventive, curative, and rehabilitative services to maximize health and well-being. It integrates care when more than one health problem exists, and deals with the context in which illness exists and influences people's responses to their health problems. It is care that organizes and rationalizes the deployment of all resources, basic as well as specialized, directed at promoting, maintaining, and improving health.

The *ideal* primary care environment is one that provides classic "comprehensive care" (Reader & Soave, 1976). In terms that still apply, Dr. John Knowles defined the latter a conference held in 1964 (1965, p. 73):

> Comprehensive medicine in this [ambulatory care] context means the coordination of all the various caring elements in the community with those of the medical profession by a team of individuals representing all disciplines, with all the techniques and resources available to the physician and his patient. The aim of these individuals would be to provide total care—somatic, psychic, and social—to those in need, and to study and research the expanding social and economic problems of medical care with the intent of improving the organization and provision of health services.

These are ideal, normative definitions of primary and comprehensive care. In *functional* terms, as noted in chapter 1, primary care is that care which most people need, and use, most of the time for most of their health concerns.

Functions

The primary feature of comprehensive primary care is its integrating role. When nearly all medical services were rendered by a family's general practitioner, coordination was almost automatic. Today, a primary-care doctor or team can still provide most of the care that is necessary most of the time. Complications or new problems at times will, however, require the expertise of others. Coordination can be assured if the primary provider assesses the situation, helps the patient with a proper referral, and then integrates the outcome of the referral into the patient's ongoing care.

This "gatekeeper" function of the primary provider prevents fragmentation and the hit-or-miss nature of self-referral to subspecialists and promotes comprehensive care, for the patient as a whole person, not merely a set of parts (Somers, 1983). In this sense, the gatekeeper function of the primary-care practitioner can only benefit the patient.

In the managed care era, however, the term "gatekeeper" has taken on a second meaning representing the second function of the primary-care physician under managed care: to monitor, regulate, and control the utilization of medical and related services by the MCO's (no longer each individual physician's) patients. Thus a fiscal responsibility has now been added to the task list of the primary-care physician. It is a responsibility the physician has to the payor for the patient's care that may on occasion conflict with the responsibility the physician has for the care of the patient. In some MCOs, managed care physicians receive monetary bonuses for holding down use of services by their patients. For more on this subject, see chapter 8.

For achieving the best in primary care (and indeed for all of medicine), as Dr. Kerr White so splendidly put it some years ago (1973, p. 362):

''One wants to avoid the confusion inherent in the encounter between the patient who implicitly says to the doctor, 'I hope you treat what I've got' and the physician who implicitly says to the patient, 'I hope you've got what I treat.' '' Another important aspect of the integrating role of comprehensive primary care is the coordination of preventive and curative services. This occurs less often than it should in much of America's clinical practice.

In contrast to the situation in many other countries, the primary-care relationship in the United States traditionally has not ended at the hospital admitting office. U.S. primary-care physicians have provided a good deal of the inpatient care. Most board-certified family practitioners, general internists, and general pediatricians in this country have hospital admitting privileges. In contrast, in most other industrialized nations primary-care physicians work only in ambulatory care offices and health centers. A separate group of specialists provides inpatient and hospital clinic care. As noted in chapter 2, however, with the growth of managed care, in the U.S. too the development of what some observers have called the ''hospitalist'' is occurring (Wachter & Goldman, 1996). It remains to be seen how far this trend of the mid-1990s will be carried.

Brief Historical Background

The primary-care concept is hardly new (M. I. Roemer, 1975). Nor has its implementation been without its champions in the United States. As far back as the 1930s it received a strong endorsement from the Committee on the Costs of Medical Care, and from many other authorities in the intervening years (Somers, 1983). In Great Britain, the concept goes back at least as far as the Dawson report of 1920 on the structure of health services (Sidel & Sidel, 1983, p. 152).

Despite these recommendations to the contrary, however, in the U.S., as physician specialization and subspecialization increased dramatically in the period following World War II, much of the ambulatory care provided in private offices and groups and in hospital outpatient departments became highly fragmented (Freymann, 1974). The need to restore continuity and coordination was recognized in the 1960s and led to a revitalization of the concept of primary care (IOM, 1978).

Many of the health services entities called Neighborhood Health Centers that developed in the 1960s and 1970s fostered the primary-care approach, as did many of the health maintenance organizations (HMOs) developed in the 1970s and 1980s (see also chapter 8). Nevertheless, in the 1990s it is still the case that many people in the United States do not have access to comprehensive primary care (Starfield, 1996). Rather they receive fragmented outpatient and inpatient services, often only after they become seriously ill. And, as Starfield has noted, the institution of primarily for-profit managed care will not necessarily remedy this situation.

Health Manpower for Primary Care

In the ideal primary-care setting an appropriately trained health professional or team provides most of the personal preventive and curative care for an individual or family over a significant period of time. In the late 1960s, a task list for the ideal primary-care system and primary-care provider was developed that is still valid (Committee on Medical Schools, 1968, p. 753):

> 1. Assessment of total patient needs before these are categorized by specialty. 2. Elaboration of a plan for meeting those needs in the order of their importance. 3. Determination of who shall meet the defined needs—physicians (generalist or specialist); non-physician members of the health care team; or social agencies. 4. Follow-up to see that needs are met. 5. Provision of such care in a continuous, coordinated and comprehensive manner. 6. Attention at each step . . . to the personal, social and family dimensions of the patient's problem. 7. The provision of health maintenance and disease prevention at the same level of importance as the provision of cure and rehabilitation.

This description of functions shows that primary care is not simply a collection of services but above all is a state of mind, to wit (Committee on Medical Schools, 1968, p. 754):

> The primary-care physician must be capable of establishing a profile of the total needs of the patient and his family. This evaluation should include social, economic, and psychological details as well as the more strictly "medical" aspects. He must know what resources are available for meeting those needs. He should then define a plan of care, deciding which parts are to be carried out by himself and which by others. The plan should have a long-range dimension. It should be understandable to the patient and his family, and it should include a follow-up on whether indicated measures have been undertaken and whether they have been effective.

In the 1990s the task list and state of mind requirements apply as well to primary-care nurse practitioners and physician assistants as to primary-care physicians (see chapter 2).

Among physicians, primary care is provided variously by family practitioners (prepared to deliver primary-care services to entire families), general pediatricians, specialists in general internal medicine, and for many women of child-bearing age by obstetrician/gynecologists. It is likely, however, that the debate over who should be doing what to whom in primary care will continue for many years to come.

Primary Care and the Health Care Delivery System

Some observers believe that the level and quality of primary-care provision serve as good markers for the quality of a nation's health care delivery system as a whole. Concerning the variation in primary-care quality among nations, Starfield has noted (1996, p. 1365):

> First, countries with better primary care tend to be countries that strive toward equity in distribution of health services and toward more equitable income distributions. Apparently, a commitment to social equity goes along with a commitment to equity in the distribution of health care resources. Second, it is not the *number* of primary care physicians, or even the *ratio* of primary care physicians to specialists, that accounts for the differential effects of the health services across those countries. Rather, the differences are a result of *how* the resources are distributed, whether or not they are organized to achieve the *functions* of primary care, and whether they clearly specify the roles and interrelationships between primary care and specialist physicians [emphasis added].

AMBULATORY CARE[1]

Definitions

Ambulatory care is personal health service given to a person who is not a bed patient in a health care institution. The term thus covers all health services other than community health services and personal health services for the institutionalized patient. The majority of physician–patient contacts in the United States occur in an ambulatory setting.

There are two principal categories of ambulatory care. The largest is that given by private physicians in solo, partnership, or private group practice, on a fee-for-service basis, and by private physicians (often the same individuals) working in one of several different types of managed care arrangements, paid either on a fee-for-service or capitation basis.

[1]In 1981, Dr. M. I. Roemer published a comprehensive review of the subject entitled *Ambulatory Health Services in America*.

The other category is that provided in organized settings. The latter is defined as a locus of medical practice with an identity independent from that of the particular individual physician(s) working in it.

This category includes, for example, hospital-based ambulatory services (e.g., clinics, emergency departments, health promotion centers), community-based hospital-type ambulatory services (e.g., outpatient surgery centers), emergency medical services systems such as those run by police and fire departments, local public health department clinics, Neighborhood Health Centers (NHCs) and Community Health Centers (CHCs), staff and group model HMOs, organized home care, Community Mental Health Centers, industrial health services, school health services, and prison health services. Unfortunately, there is not space in this book to cover all of these categories.

Utilization

In 1994 there were over 22 times as many ambulatory patient visits to nonfederally employed physicians (681 million) as there were admissions to the nonfederal short-term general or other special hospitals (AHA, 1995; Schappert, 1996). This was more than double the ratio that existed just six years previously. Americans averaged 2.6 physician visits per person annually, in the range of the annual per capita visit rates that held from 1975 through 1994 of 2.6 to 3.0.

Females made about 60% of all physician office visits, with rates higher than those of males in all the age groups other than the youngest (under 15 years) and the oldest (65 and over), in which groups the gender/visit rates were not significantly different. Visit rates tend to increase with age after the age of 24 (as one might expect, given the natural aging process and the impact it has on health and sickness status). Although in 1994, white people had about one more office visit per year than did Blacks (2.8 to 1.7), in 1981 the visit rates by ethnic group had been virtually the same (USDHHS, 1984). Thus an equalization trend that had been underway since 1964 was reversed.

The top six specialties visited were, as might be expected: general and family practice, internal medicine, pediatrics, obstetrics and gynecology, orthopedics, and ophthalmology. Together, they accounted for over 70% of all ambulatory visits. Over 80% of physician office visits were made by patients who had seen a physician on some previous occasion, whereas over 60% were made by patients returning for care of a previously treated problem. As to sources of payment, 39% of visits were covered by private indemnity insurance, close to 22% by Medicare, close to 22% by an HMO, over 12% by the patient directly, and almost 10% by Medicaid.

The top six reasons for making an office visit to a physician were: general medical exam, progress visit, cough, routine prenatal exam, and symptoms referable to the throat. More specific diagnosis-based reasons for a visit, such as depression, ear infection, vision dysfunction, skin rash, back symptoms, knee symptoms appear further down on the list. Except for depression (at 2.2%), each of the above diagnoses accounted for less than 2.0% of all visits.

Hospital Outpatient Departments

Introduction

For a variety of historical reasons, traditionally most American hospitals have focused the bulk of their efforts and activities on inpatients who are acutely ill and confined to bed (Freymann, 1974). Hospitals also have had to deal with a variety of other types of patients, however. Most of them are known as outpatients.

Hospital outpatients require either immediate treatment for an acute and often serious illness or injury, or ongoing care for a more routine matter. Very often the services of the latter type are similar to those needed by patients who attend physicians' ambulatory care offices. In theory at least, there are two categories of hospital ambulatory services, corresponding to the two categories of patient needs: emergency services, provided by emergency rooms or departments (EDs), and clinic services or outpatient departments (OPDs).

In the real world, overlap between the two categories of patient and service is increasing. Patients, hospital staff, and hospital administration, separately and together, are sometimes confused about the differences in role and function of the two divisions. All three groups sometimes have trouble deciding which patients should go where for what.

The original intended functions of hospital emergency service units were to take care of people acutely ill or injured, particularly with life-threatening or potentially life-threatening problems that required immediate attention with personnel, and/or equipment not found in private practitioners' offices; and to offer the availability of prompt hospitalization if needed. Most hospitals have found it desirable or necessary (legally required in many states) to provide such services.

Traditionally, it was easier for hospitals to determine that emergency services should be provided than that clinic services should be. One reason for this was that insurance carriers were more likely to reimburse hospitals for emergency services than for clinic services. Under managed care, and with the steadily increasing number of Americans who have no or inadequate health care payment coverage, this situation is changing. In fact, the use of EDs for nonpreapproved, nonurgent care by persons covered by an MCO has created a major cost-containment problem for the managed care industry. In an increasing number of instances, the MCO is refusing to pay the hospital for such care.

Historical Background

In the 19th century, clinic service was part of the function of most hospitals serving the poor in urban areas (Freymann, 1974). By 1916, 495 hospitals had clinics, often serving an educational as well as a charitable function (M. I. Roemer, 1981). The original purpose of some of the hospitals built during this period was to provide special services to meet needs brought on by a rapidly changing world. For example, in 1908 the Goshen (NY) Emergency Hospital was established. Its creation was stimulated by the building of one of New York State's early trunk highways, Route 17. The road went through the center of the village of Goshen. Traffic accidents occurred with increasing frequency; *ergo* the hospital was needed.

Both the voluntaries and the local government hospitals provided free-clinic care to the poor. In most cases, however, the voluntaries established clinics on their premises only grudgingly, as they were likely to be used by nonpaying patients. Because the voluntary hospital medical staffs consisted primarily of physicians practicing privately in the community, voluntary hospital OPDs, originally staffed on a rotating basis by the members of the hospital medical staff working there without pay, were much more important in setting the style for the organization of medical practice than were those of the local government hospitals. (For the contemporary staffing arrangements, see below.)

Hospital Outpatient Department Utilization

During 1994, over 66 million visits were made to hospital OPDs in nonfederal short-term general and other special hospitals, over 25 visits per 100 persons per year (Lipkind, 1996). Paralleling the general ambulatory patient usage figures, females had higher visit rates than males. In contrast, the visit rate for Blacks was higher than that for Whites in all age categories except under 15 and 75 and over. Medicaid and private indemnity insurance were the two most common payment sources. The three most common reasons for visiting were "progress visit," general medical exam, and routine prenatal exam, whereas the three most common diagnoses were normal pregnancy, essential hypertension, and diabetes mellitus. Sixty-five percent of all OPD visits resulted in an appointment for a return visit.

Hospital OPD Organization and Staffing

Although not all clinics are found in teaching hospitals (those affiliated with medical schools), they are the archetype. Given the way contemporary medical education is structured, the teaching hospitals found that the best way of organizing OPDs to provide opportunities for teaching and research was to have many disease-, organ-, or organ-system-specific clinics (Freymann, 1974). Typically the contemporary teaching hospital has three groups of clinics: medical, surgical, and other.

The medical clinics, of which a family practice unit or a general medical clinic approximating the function of the general internist may be a part, include, for example, cardiology, neurology, dermatology, allergy, gastroenterology, and so on. General surgery, orthopedics, urology, plastic surgery, and the like comprise the surgical clinic group. Included in the third, ''catch-all'' group are pediatrics and the pediatric subspecialties, obstetrics–gynecology and its subspecialties, and ''others'' such as rehabilitation medicine.

The larger teaching hospitals often have over 100 different specialty and subspecialty clinics. Thus, a hospital-based physician working in the usual hospital-clinic organization can concentrate on diabetes, peripheral vascular disease, or stroke in her or his teaching and/or research. This is useful for the provider focusing on a particular disease or condition. It may also be helpful to the patient who has a single disease or problem of a rather complex or unusual nature. But this may be detrimental for the patient with multiple problems who may find her or himself divided between multiple clinics, with no one physician coordinating this person's care and providing an overview of the patient as a person rather than a collection of organ systems.

There are five functional categories of physician staff in teaching hospital clinics. First, it was formerly very common for the hospital's ''voluntary'' attending medical staff to draw clinic duty as part of the obligation incurred for the granting of admitting privileges for their private patients, at no cost to themselves. This is still the case in some institutions.

Second, in the 1980s many medical schools became increasingly dependent on the financial support of physician income earned in the clinics. The money is derived primarily from third-party payors (see chapter 5). Thus, as noted, many clinics are now staffed by medical-school faculty whose work there generates both some of their own income and money for the school's general fund. The management system for dividing this income between the physicians and the institution providing the space and supporting staff is usually called the ''clinical-practice plan.'' Depending on the particular arrangements, for some physicians the medical school hospitals have become more rather than less attractive places in which to work.

Third, to carry out teaching, supervisory, and research functions, the hospital may assign full-time salaried inpatient physicians, usually the more junior ones, to the clinics. Fourth, house staff (physicians in postmedical school, graduate specialty training, the interns and residents), usually draw significant clinic duty from time to time throughout the course of their training. Finally, for clinics with many patient visits, hospitals may hire outside physicians exclusively to work on a sessional or part-time salaried basis.

Some Problems Faced by Clinic Patients

The basic contradiction in hospital ambulatory services is clear. On the one hand there are the teaching and research needs of specialty-oriented providers. On the other there are the needs of patients with either ordinary problems or several different problems requiring the care of several specialties. This situation is not new; neither are professional recognition of it and the recommendations for correcting it. Over 30 years ago, in 1964, at a conference on ‘‘The Expanding Role of Ambulatory Services in Hospitals and Health Departments’’ held at the New York Academy of Medicine, Cecil Sheps, M.D. (1965, p. 148), said:

> As I sat through the sessions yesterday and today I had a persistent feeling of *deja vu*. I possess a book written by Michael M. Davis and published in 1927 [*Clinics, Hospitals and Health Centers*, New York: Harper]. In it there is quoted a statement prepared in 19*14* that describes the purpose of an out-patient department just as clearly as anything said at this conference; that the focus must be on the patient, that care must be organized around the patient, and that the hospital must take the community as its venue and not simply the patients who come to it [emphasis added].

An echo of this recommendation was found in John Gordon Freymann’s ‘‘mission-oriented hospital’’ concepts from the 1970s (see the previous chapter). The 1990s version of what Dr. Davis was talking about in 1927 is called community-oriented primary care (Madison, 1983; Mullan, 1982; Mullan & Connor, 1982; Nutting et al., 1985). Its major elements are as follows:

1. The clinical practice of comprehensive primary medical care.
2. The use of applied epidemiology in practice planning.
3. Community involvement in program planning.
4. The use of data gathered in practice operations in a feedback loop.

5. Continuing surveillance of community health status and needs.

The model can be used in any medical practice, whether solo, group, or hospital-based. The principal problem is not conceptual; the ideas have been with us for many years. The difficulty is in implementation: to this day there are only a few institutions that approach the ideal as previously set forth.

Hospital Emergency Services

During 1994 Americans made over 93 million visits to emergency departments (EDs) in nonfederal short-term hospitals, about 36 visits per 100 persons per year (Stussman, 1996). Persons 75 and older had a higher visit rate than persons in all of the other age categories. A quarter of all ED visits were made by children under 15. Blacks had a higher visit rate than Whites. Over 40% of all visits were for the treatment of injuries, with more than one third of them occurring in the home. Ear infection was the single most common principle diagnosis for an ED visit. Medications were subscribed in over 75% of all ED visits.

The hospital ED serves a variety of functions. First, it provides care to critically ill and injured patients, of course. Second, in many hospitals it also serves as a secondary, well-equipped private physician's office. There, staff physicians can see their own patients who require more sophisticated care than that available in the doctor's private offices. Third, EDs are a source of patient admissions to the hospital.

A fourth role that has become increasingly important in the years since World War II is the provision of care to persons who are not injured or critically ill, but who have not seen or cannot see their private physician, or who find that their regular clinic is not open when needed, or who find that their regular or covering HMO-assigned primary-care "gatekeeper" physician is not available or not conveniently available when needed, or they need care when they are geographically "out of region."

In terms that still apply, back in 1966 Weinerman et al. (p. 1040) defined three categories of patients presenting themselves to emergency units:

1. *Nonurgent*: Condition does not require the resources of an emergency service; referral for routine medical care may or may not be needed; disorder is nonacute or minor in severity.
2. *Urgent*: Condition requires medical attention within the period of a few hours; there is a possible danger to the patient if medically unattended; disorder is acute but not necessarily severe.

3. *Emergent*: Condition requires immediate medical attention; time delay is harmful to patient; disorder is acute and potentially threatening to life or function.

Of course, these definitions are made from the professional perspective. Many patients do not make the kinds of distinctions health professionals make. Many voluntary visits to emergency rooms are for conditions that are neither "urgent" nor "emergent" from a medical viewpoint. Nevertheless, most patients presenting themselves for care to EDs do so because, regardless of how their problem might be classified by a provider, they feel the need for immediate attention and cannot find care elsewhere. Whatever the patient's problem is, it is distressing to him or her. Such patients, however, load emergency departments with responsibilities with which they are not equipped to deal.

In the view of many analysts, several of whom are quoted throughout the pages of this book, the solution must be found outside the walls of the hospital. It must encompass an integrated system of medical care for the entire community assuring availability of appropriate medical care at all hours and to all classes of the population. Thus we come full circle back to the definitions of comprehensive and community-oriented primary care reviewed at the beginning of this chapter, to the visions of Michael Davis, John Knowles, and John Gorden Freymann, and to the problems of availability and accessibility in a system in which, for openers, over 40 million people have no coverage for health care costs.

Hospital Ambulatory Services Outside the Walls of the Hospital

From the 1980s onward, hospitals have been developing community-based facilities to provide services that have traditionally required inpatient stays, but with advances in medical practice and technology can now safely be provided on an outpatient basis (Anderson, 1990; Ermann & Gabel, 1985; Podolsky, 1996). These facilities include, for example: satellite OPDs (that may simply be a set of separate specialty clinics à la many hospitals, or may be more like a community health center), comprehensive diagnostic centers (for lab, X-ray, and related functions), "surgi-centers" where surgery that can be safely performed on an outpatient basis is done.

Nonhospital-Based Emergency Medical Services

Nonhospital-based emergency medical services (EMS) have three principal components (R. Roemer et al., 1975): (1) ambulance services and emergency prehospital care, (2) emergency medical care provided at the hospital, and (3) disaster medical services.

Federal EMS legislation from the 1970s identified 15 components of a functioning emergency medical services system (Hoffer, 1979): provision of a labor force, training of personnel, communications, transportation, facilities, critical-care units, use of public-safety agencies, consumer participation, accessibility to care, transfer of patients, standard medical record keeping, consumer information and education, independent review and evaluation, disaster linkage, and mutual-aid agreements.

A principal goal for EMS program developers has been to provide the whole nation with a network of coordinated emergency care dispatch centers, using the uniform emergency telephone number 911. That goal has yet to be achieved.

Ambulance design has progressed significantly. Historically, ambulance services developed from a for-profit enterprise established by funeral directors. In this system, sometimes the same vehicle served more than one purpose, on occasion consecutively. Beginning in the 1970s, specialized, sometimes very highly equipped vehicles, manned by well-trained personnel, began to make their appearance, and are now quite common in many areas of the country.

Given that traumatic injury is among the leading causes of death in the productive age groups, and given that early attention following traumatic injury can often be lifesaving, the development of a national trauma-services system is especially important. This prospect is in the early stages of development. As Bazzoli et al. (1995, p. 395) point out:

> From 1988 to 1993, the number of states meeting one set of criteria for a complete trauma system increased from two to five. The most common deficiency in establishing trauma systems was failure to limit the number of designated trauma centers based on community need. . . . State and regional organizations have accomplished a great deal but still have substantial work ahead in developing comprehensive trauma systems.

Public Health Agency Clinics

In many parts of the United States local government provides ambulatory personal health services both in public hospitals and other venues (see also chapter 6). Local health departments operate an array of special clinics, focusing primarily on the prevention of disease.

Important among their services are clinics for tuberculosis control (often providing treatment as well as case-finding services), child health (where immunizations, examinations, and education on child rearing are provided), prenatal care, sexually transmitted disease control, and mental health problems. In recent years, some public health agencies have broadened the scope of their services to include such elements as family planning, chronic disease detection, and general primary (disease treatment) care. Precisely how much care is provided is not known. Although there are over 2,000 local health department units providing some kind of care, public health services are not a major factor in the overall ambulatory care picture.

The provision of personal disease treatment service by local health departments has been a subject of controversy ever since the practice began in the 19th century (Rosen, 1971; Winslow, 1929). Battles over the role of local health departments were especially fierce during the 192Os, when some local health departments developed plans to expand their general disease treatment services (Myers et al., 1968; Rosen, 1971; Winslow, 1929). The efforts of the organized representatives of American physicians to stop these developments generally met with success (see also below). To this day, most personal services of local health departments are usually limited to those areas in which private physicians are either not very interested (routine well-baby examinations), not especially competent (treatment, case finding, and contact investigation for sexually transmitted diseases and tuberculosis), or not available (primary care in underserved areas).

In the current era there has been a diminution of organized medicine's opposition to the involvement of local health departments in the provision of direct medical services to the poor. Some hard-pressed urban and suburban health departments have done this, especially where access to public hospital services is limited or nonexistent.

Neighborhood and Community Health Centers

In the late 1960s and early 1970s a phenomenon called the Neighborhood Health Center movement emerged on the American health care scene. The NHC was based on the concepts of full-time salaried physician staffing, multidisciplinary team-health-care practice, and community involvement in both policymaking and facility operations (Davis & Schoen, 1978; Zwick, 1974). The movement was strongly stimulated by a federal agency called the Office of Economic Opportunity (OEO). It was the lead agency for the "war on poverty" conducted by President Lyndon Johnson's Administration in the period between 1964 and 1968.

The Neighborhood Health Center movement was the basis of a rallying cry for change both in the content and the availability of health services for the poor, a focus for the way "to do things right." The NHCs aimed to provide, mainly for poor people, one-stop shopping for comprehensive ambulatory care—a full range of preventive and rehabilitative as well as treatment services that were acceptable, affordable, and of high quality. The NHC program aimed to bring such services to many more people than had access to any kind of health care at the time.

The NHCs also aimed to intervene in the cycle of poverty, by providing jobs and skills/career development opportunities for the residents of the communities they served. The movement did not meet with overwhelming success, to say the least, in terms of patient visits provided, for example. Conceptually it was very important, however. For example, its basic health service precepts have been vital to the Community-Oriented Primary Care (COPC) model mentioned above (Mullan & Conner, 1982).

The NHC did not represent an entirely new concept in the United States. The 19th-century free-standing urban "dispensary" was an early general ambulatory care center that primarily served the poor. Although it was organized differently, it performed some functions similar to that of the modern NHC or CHC (the NHC's successor). Health department ambulatory care programs developed during the last quarter of the 19th century had some elements that would also appear later in NHCs, such as districting and, on occasion, comprehensiveness (Rosen, 1971).

During the period from 1920 to 1923 Herman Biggs, M.D., then Commissioner of Health of New York State, tried vigorously, but quite unsuccessfully, to get the state and local health departments away from the categorical disease approach and into the business of delivering comprehensive health services (Winslow, 1929). As noted above, organized medicine successfully fought against the broad establishment of any health care delivery model not based on private practice (except for service to the very poor).

The experience with prepaid group practice (PPGP) in the 1930s, 1940s, and 1950s (see also chapter 8) influenced the development of the NHC movement of the 1960s and 1970s (Light & Brown, 1967). With varying degrees of vigor and success, the NHCs attempted to make multidisciplinary group practice work. As well as physicians and nurses, they employed social workers, "neighborhood health workers" (usually people from the area served, specially trained by the NHC with a combination of basic nursing and social service skills), and sometimes lawyers, all on salary. These folks were combined into a health care team to help patients deal with their social and medical problems.

At the movement's peak in the early 1970s, there were an estimated 200 NHCs nationally (*Health PAC Bulletin*, 1972). In the mid-1970s, the Nixon and Ford administrations more narrowly defined the scope of the NHC program and renamed it the Community Health Center program. The CHCs, which included many of the original NHCs, were to concentrate on the delivery of primary-care services. They were to deemphasize other

NHC roles, such as providing employment opportunities and training programs, stimulating social and economic development in their communities, and concerning themselves with community-wide as well as personal health problems.

By the early 1980s, there were over 800 CHCs serving over 4.5 million people (Sardell, 1983), a remarkable resurgence for a program that received little publicity. By the early 1990s (Starfield, 1992), there were 540 CHCs with a total of 2,000 locations serving close to 6 million poor people in all 50 states, the District of Columbia, and the major U.S. territories. As of fiscal year 1996, there were over 600 community and migrant worker comprehensive primary-care systems with over 1,600 sites, providing care for about 8 million people, close to 80% of whom were either Medicaid recipients or uninsured (HRSA, 1990).

The CHCs are supported primarily by federal grant funds, plus third-party reimbursements and private fees paid on a sliding scale. Close to half of CHC physicians are drawn from the National Health Service Corps, a program that provides financial aid for medical school tuition in return for a commitment to serve in a program of the CHC type for a specified period of time after medical school graduation.

Industrial Health Service Units

A wide range of industrial health hazards exist, from traumatic injury to occupational exposure to harmful substances (e.g., silica, asbestos, lead). The number of "in-plant" health units in the United States is not known, but there are thousands of them. In small plants (less than 100 workers), health services are ordinarily quite rudimentary. They are often limited to a first-aid box and arrangements with some local health facility to which injured workers may be sent. Very large plants (with more than 2,500 workers) usually have some systematic in-plant health service. Customarily it is staffed with trained industrial nurses and part-time or full-time physicians. In a few firms, in-plant health services are comprehensive, providing employees with complete medical care for all disorders, whether or not they are job connected.

The long-term trend in American industry is toward the greater concentration of production in fewer large corporations. Although at one time it seemed that concentration might enhance the prospects for improving occupational health programs, in the latter half of the 1980s, there were actually reductions in service in many large corporations in the name of cost savings (D. Parkinson, personal communication, October 25, 1990).

A relatively recent development in occupational health is the "worksite health promotion" program (Scofield, 1990). A national authority on worksite wellness/health promotion programs, Dr. Michael O'Donnell, defined health promotion as (O'Donnell & Harris, 1994, p. xi):

> The science and art of helping people change their lifestyle to move toward a state of optimal health. Optimal health is defined as a balance of physical, emotional, social, spiritual and intellectual health. Lifestyle change can be facilitated through a combination of efforts to enhance awareness, change behavior and create environments that support good health practices. Of the three, supporting environments will probably have the greatest impact in producing lasting changes.

As of the mid-90s, more than 80% of businesses employing more than 50 workers had some kind of health-promotion program (O'Donnell & Harris, 1994). According to James Terborg (1986, p. 225):

> Worksite health promotion consists of an ongoing series of activities funded or endorsed by the organization that are designed to promote the adoption of personal behavior and corporate practices that are conducive to employee fitness, health, and wellness. Instruction [and often the opportunity/facility for engaging in the activity] is typically provided at the worksite in areas such as exercise, strength training, weight loss, smoking cessation, stress management, blood pressure monitoring and control, and nutrition.

Worksite health promotion or wellness programs can operate on three levels: enhancing employee awareness of the several factors in health and how they can be striven for, assisting employees in actually making changes, and developing the workplace environment(s) conducive to health (O'Donnell & Harris, 1994). There is some evidence that the provision of such services by companies is cost-effective (Kamen, 1995; Shephard, 1986).

School Health Clinics

In 1990 there were over 64.5 million students in over 88,000 primary and secondary schools, colleges, and universities (USBoC, 1995). Almost all of the educational institutions provide some type of organized, ambulatory health service. About one half of the school health services are run by local health departments, the balance being run by boards of education, on their own (25%) or in cooperation with the local health department.

Very little disease treatment is done in school health programs. Usually carried out by school nurses, the work of most of these programs is confined to case finding and prevention for certain chronic or epidemic diseases, for example, screening for vision and hearing difficulties and providing immunizations. Referrals are made to physicians for diagnosis and treatment, should they be indicated. College and university health services are more likely to provide general diagnostic and treatment care. Some pay special attention to mental and substance abuse problems.

Home Care and Hospice

According to Strahan (1996):

> Home health care is provided to individuals and families in their place of residence to promote, maintain, or restore health or to maximize the level of independence while minimizing the effects of disability and illness, including terminal illness. These agencies are often referred to today as "hospitals with walls" because advances in technology allow dozens of complex illnesses, once treated almost exclusively in the hospital, to be treated at home.
>
> Hospice care is defined as a program of palliative and supportive care services that provides physical, psychological, social, and spiritual care for dying persons, their families, and other loved ones. Hospice services are available in both the home and inpatient settings. [p. 1]

In 1994 there were an estimated 10,900 home health care and hospice agencies in the United States, a 30% increase in the number of agencies since 1992. About 9,800 of these were home health agencies. Overall, 44% of the agencies were privately owned, whereas 37% were not for profit. Of the hospice agencies, 90% were not for profit. Of the total patient population, 59% of home health care and 86% of hospice patients were being taken care of by not-for-profit agencies.

In that year (1994), there were about 1.9 million persons receiving home health care. They were predominately elderly, female, White, and married or widowed. The major medical diagnoses for this group were heart disease (53%), stroke, hypertension, and diabetes. The predominant diagnosis for the hospice group was, not surprisingly, cancer (59%). Next came diseases of the circulatory system. Patients with a diagnosis related to infection with the human immunodeficiency virus (HIV) accounted for 3% of hospice patients in 1994.

CONCLUSIONS

The bulk of the need for medical care and for the provision of health services occurs in the ambulatory setting. In the U.S., a disproportionate share of health care resources are devoted to inpatient care, both acute and long term. If, overall, health care is to be improved in the United States, this imbalance needs to be addressed. Furthermore, given the current profile of disease and disability in the United States, it is obvious that significant improvements in the health of the American people could be achieved by the widespread implementation of known health-promotive/disease-preventive measures, in the ambulatory setting (USDHHS, 1990, 1995). This is a central element of comprehensive primary care.

As stated at the outset of this chapter, primary care goes with ambulatory care like ice cream goes with apple pie (neither of which is unhealthy if eaten only occasionally). Historically, there is movement in the right direction. Much remains to be done.

REFERENCES

AHA (American Hospital Association). *Hospital stat, 1995–6*. Chicago: Author, 1995.

Anderson, H. Out-patient care: A nationwide revolution. *Hospitals*, August 5, 1990, p. 28.

Bazzoli, G. J. et al. Progress in the development of trauma systems in the United States. *Journal of the American Medical Association, 273,* 395, 1995.

Committee on Medical Schools of the Association of American Medical Colleges in Relation to Training for Family Practice. Planning for comprehensive and continuing care of patients through education. *Journal of Medical Education, 43,* 751, 1968.

Davis, G. S. Introduction: Managed health care primer. In National Health Lawyers Association, *The insider's guide to managed care*. Washington, DC: National Health Lawyers Association, 1990.

Davis, K., & Schoen, C. *Health and the War on Poverty*. Washington, DC: The Brookings Institution, 1978.

Ermann, D., & Gabel, J. The changing face of American health care: Multihospital systems, emergency centers, and surgery centers. *Medical Care, 23,* 401, 1985.

Freymann, J. G. *The American health care system: Its genesis and trajectory*. New York: Medcom Press, 1974.

Health PAC Bulletin. NENA: Community control in a bind. June 1972.

HRSA (Health Resources and Services Administration). *A profile*. Washington, DC: US Public Health Service, April 1990.

Hoffer, E. P. Emergency medical services, 1979. *New England Journal of Medicine, 301,* 1118, 1979.

IOM (Institute of Medicine). *A manpower policy for primary health care*. Washington, DC: National Academy of Sciences, 1978.

Kamen, R. L. *Worksite health promotion economics: Consensus and analysis*. Champaign, IL: Human Kinetics, 1995.

Knowles, J. H. The role of the hospital: The ambulatory clinic. *Bulletin of the New York Academy of Medicine, 41*(2), 68, 1965.

Light, H. L., & Brown, H. J. The Gouverneur Health Services Program: An historical view. *Milbank Memorial Fund Quarterly, 45,* 375, 1967.

Lipkind, K. L. National hospital ambulatory medical care survey: 1994, outpatient department summary. *Advance Data*, No. 276, June 11, 1996.

Madison, D. L. The case for community-oriented primary care. *Journal of the American Medical Association, 249,* 1279, 1983.

Medical Benefits. The interstudy edge. *6*(11), 1, 1989.

Mullan, F. Community-oriented primary care. *New England Journal of Medicine, 307,* 1076, 1982.

Mullan, F., & Conner, E. (Eds.). *Community-oriented primary care—Conference Proceedings*. Washington, DC: National Academy Press, 1982.

Myers, B. A. et al. The medical care activities of local health units. *Public Health Reports, 83,* 757, 1968.

Nutting, P. A. et al. Community-oriented primary care in the United States. *Journal of the American Medical Association, 253*, 1763, 1985.

O'Donnell, M., & Harris, J. (Eds.). *Health promotion in the workplace* (2nd ed.). Albany, NY: Delmar Publishers, 1994.

Podolsky, D. Breaking down the walls. *U.S. News and World Report*, August 12, 1996, p. 61.

Reader, G. G., & Soave, R. Comprehensive care revisited. *Milbank Memorial Fund Quarterly: Health and Society*, Fall, 1976, p. 391.

Roemer, M. I. From poor beginnings, the growth of primary care. *Hospitals*, March 1, 1975, p. 38.

Roemer, M. I. *Ambulatory health services in America*. Gaithersburg, MD: Aspen, 1981.

Roemer, R. et al. *Planning urban health services: From jungle to system*. New York: Springer Publishing Co., 1975.

Rosen, G. The first neighborhood health center movement—Its rise and fall. *American Journal of Public Health, 61,* 1620, 1971.

Ruby, G. et al. Definitions of primary care (staff paper). Washington, DC: Institute of Medicine, 1977.

Sardell, A. Neighborhood health centers and community-based care: Federal policy from 1965 to 1982. *Journal of Public Health Policy, 4,* 484, 1983.

Schappert, S. M. National Ambulatory Medical Care Survey: 1994 summary. *Advance Data*, No. 273, April 10, 1996.

Scofield, M. E. (Ed.). *Worksite health promotion.* Philadelphia, PA: Hanley & Belfus, 1990.

Shephard, R. J. *Economic benefits of enhanced fitness.* Champaign, IL: Human Kinetics Publishers, 1986.

Sheps, C. G. Conference summary and the road ahead. *Bulletin of the New York Academy of Medicine, 41*(1), 146, 1965.

Sidel, V. W., & Sidel, R. *A healthy state* (revised). New York: Pantheon Books, 1983.

Somers, A. R. And who shall be the gatekeeper? The role of the primary physician in the health care delivery system. *Inquiry, 20,* 301, 1983.

Starfield, B. *Primary care.* New York: Oxford University Press, 1992.

Starfield, B. Public health and primary care: A framework for proposed linkages. *American Journal of Public Health, 86,* 1365, 1996.

Strahan, G. W. An overview of home health and hospice care patients: 1994 National Home and Hospice Care Survey. *Advance Data*, No. 274, April 24, 1996.

Stussman, B. J. National Hospital Ambulatory Medical Care Survey: 1994 emergency department summary. *Advance Data*, No. 275, May 1996.

Terborg, J. R. Health promotion at the worksite: A research challenge for personnel and human resources management. *Research in Personnel and Human Resources Management, 4,* 225, 1986.

USBoC (U.S. Bureau of the Census). *Statistical abstract of the United States: 1995* (115th ed.). Washington, DC: U.S.G.P.O., 1995.

USDHHS (U.S. Department of Health and Human Services). *Health United States, 1984*. Pub. No. (PHS) 85-1232. Washington, DC: U.S.G.P.O., 1984.

USDHHS. *Healthy people 2000.* Washington, DC: U.S.G.P.O., 1990.

USDHHS. *Healthy people 2000: Midcourse review and 1995 revisions.* Washington, DC: U.S.G.P.O., 1995.

Wachter, R. M., & Goldman, L. The emerging role of ''hospitalists'' in the American health care system. *New England Journal of Medicine, 335,* 514, 1996.

Weinerman, E. R. Problems and perspectives of group practice. *Bulletin of the New York Academy of Medicine* (2nd Series), *44*, 1423, 1968.

White, K. L. Organization and delivery of personal health services—Public policy issues. *Milbank Memorial Fund Quarterly*, January 1968. Reprinted in J. B. McKinlay (Ed.), *Politics and Law in Health Care Policy*, New York: Prodist, 1973.

Winslow, C.-E. A. *The life of Herman Biggs.* Philadelphia, PA: Lea and Febiger, 1929.

Zwick, D. I. Some accomplishments and findings of neighborhood health centers. *Milbank Memorial Fund Quarterly*, October 1972. Reprinted in I. K. Zola & J. B. McKinlay (Eds.), *Organizational issues in the delivery of health services.* New York: Prodist, 1974.

Chapter 5
Financing

All the money used to pay for health care comes from the people. Most of it goes to pay the institutional and individual providers for their services. Third parties[1] handling money transfers retain a certain percentage of the money transferred. As noted previously on several occasions, with the growth of for-profit managed care, an increasing portion of health care dollars are going to provide profits for the increasing number of for-profit managed care organizations (MCOs).

In the first chapter we described the five major components of the health care delivery system: health care institutions, personnel, "health commodities" firms, education/research institutions, and the financing system. The latter is the component that makes it possible for the first four to interact with each other and produce what we call "health care."

Because the United States lacks a single national health care payment system covering everybody, just how the money gets from the people to the providers has become a very complicated matter. This chapter describes the basics of health care financing and the system that handles its functions: How much money is spent, where the money comes from (e.g., direct out-of-pocket payments, a private insurance company or an MCO), what it is spent on (e.g., fees to individual providers, payments to hospitals), and how it is paid out to the providers (e.g., item of service, per unit of care, capitation).

HOW MUCH IS SPENT[2]

In 1988 health care payments totaled about $540 billion, an increase of 10.4% over the previous year (ONCE, 1990). The 1988 overall inflation

[1]A "third party" is an entity other than the patient or the care provider, such as a health insurance company or a managed care organization (MCO).

rate was 4.1% (USBoC, 1990). About 89% of total expenditures went for personal health services. The balance was paid for research, facilities construction, program administration, private health insurance administration, and public health services.

In 1994, just 6 years later, health care payments totaled about $950 billion, an increase of 6.4% over the previous year (Levit et al., 1996), and about *75% higher* than the total in 1988. The 1994 overall inflation rate was about 3.5%. Changing little since 1988, about 88% of total expenditures went for personal health services. As in previous years, the balance was paid for research, facilities construction, program administration, private health insurance administration and profits, and public health services.

In 1994 health care spending accounted for 13.7% of the gross domestic product (GDP). That figure is about 38% higher than the percentage of the GDP spent by the country with the next highest spending rate—Canada (USBoC, 1995). But, Canada has a comprehensive national health insurance program (see chapter 9).

In both absolute and relative terms national health expenditures have grown considerably over the years (see Table 5.1). Between 1960 and 1994 national health care payments increased over 35-fold in current dollars, 4.4 times in constant dollars. In 1960 health care expenditures accounted for only 5.3% of the gross national product (GNP), in contrast with the 13.6% of the GDP spent in 1994. Between 1970 and 1991 the annual rate of increase in health care expenditures was constantly in the double-digit range, even when inflation and the GNP/GDP growth rate were not. Why this happened is a matter of much cogitation and controversy.

In the 1990s, with the advent of managed care and its downward pressure on both physician and hospital usage, a brake has been put on health care cost increases, at least for the time being: the rates of increase were 9.4%, 6.3%, and 5.7%, respectively for 1992, 1993, and 1994. A considerable part of the constant upward trend in U.S. health care spending has been caused by factors other than simple utilization, however, such as the ever-intensifying use of expensive technology-based diagnostic and procedural interventions, especially at the beginning and the end of life (Franks & Clancy, 1992). Thus, it remains to be seen for how long the expenditure increase rate will remain at a relatively modest level (although still above the general rate of inflation).

---

[2]The data presented in this chapter are drawn largely from the articles "National health expenditures, 1988," by the Office of National Cost Estimates, *Health Care Financing Review*, 1990, *11*(4), pp. 1–54, abbreviated "ONCE" in the text references, and K. R. Levit et al., "National health expenditures, 1994," *Health Care Financing Review*, 1996, *17*(3), pp. 205–242.

TABLE 5.1 National Health Expenditures Aggregate and Per Capita Amounts, Percent Distribution, and Average Annual Percent Growth, by Source of Funds: Selected Years 1960–94

Item	1960	1970	1975	1980	1985	1990	1991	1992	1993	1994
	Amount in Billions									
National Health Expenditures	$26.9	$73.2	$130.7	$247.2	$428.2	$697.5	$761.3	$833.6	$892.3	$949.4
Private	20.2	45.5	75.7	142.5	253.9	413.1	441.0	477.0	505.1	528.6
Public	6.6	27.7	55.0	104.8	174.3	284.3	320.3	356.5	387.2	420.8
Federal	2.9	17.8	36.4	72.0	123.3	195.8	224.4	254.8	278.5	303.6
State and Local	3.7	9.9	18.6	32.8	51.0	88.5	95.8	101.8	108.6	117.2
	Number in Millions									
U.S. Population[1]	190.1	214.8	224.5	235.1	246.9	259.5	262.3	265.1	267.9	270.5
	Amount in Billions									
Gross Domestic Product	$527	$1,036	$1,631	$2,784	$4,181	$5,744	$5,917	$6,244	$6,550	$6,931
	Per Capita Amount									
National Health Expenditures	$141	$341	$582	$1,052	$1,735	$2,688	$2,902	$3,144	$3,331	$3,510
Private	106	212	337	606	1,029	1,592	1,681	1,799	1,886	1,954
Public	35	129	245	446	706	1,096	1,221	1,345	1,445	1,556
Federal	15	83	162	306	499	754	856	961	1,040	1,122
State and Local	20	46	83	140	207	341	365	384	406	433

Item	1960	1970	1975	1980	1985	1990	1991	1992	1993	1994
					Percent Distribution					
National Health Expenditures	100.0	100.0	100.0	100.0	100.0	100.0	100.0	100.0	100.0	100.0
Private	75.2	62.2	57.9	57.6	59.3	59.2	57.9	57.2	56.6	55.7
Public	24.8	37.8	42.1	42.4	40.7	40.8	42.1	42.8	43.4	44.3
Federal	10.9	24.3	27.8	29.1	28.8	28.1	29.5	30.6	31.2	32.0
State and Local	13.9	13.5	14.2	13.3	11.9	12.7	12.6	12.2	12.2	12.3
					Percent of Gross Domestic Product					
National Health Expenditures	5.1	7.1	8.0	8.9	10.2	12.1	12.9	13.3	13.6	13.7
					Average Annual Percent Growth from Previous Year Shown					
National Health Expenditures	—	10.6	12.3	13.6	11.6	10.2	9.1	9.5	7.0	6.4
Private	—	8.5	10.7	13.5	12.3	10.2	6.7	8.2	5.9	4.7
Public	—	15.3	14.7	13.7	10.7	10.3	12.7	11.3	8.6	8.7
Federal	—	19.8	15.4	14.6	11.4	9.7	14.6	13.5	9.3	9.0
State and Local	—	10.2	13.5	12.0	9.2	11.6	8.3	6.2	6.7	7.9
U.S. Population	—	1.2	0.9	0.9	1.0	1.0	1.1	1.1	1.0	1.0
Gross Domestic Product	—	7.0	9.5	11.3	8.5	6.6	3.0	5.5	4.9	5.8

[1]July 1 Social Security area population estimates for each year, 1960–94.
NOTE: Numbers and percents may not add to totals because of rounding.
SOURCE: Health Care Financing Administration, Office of the Actuary: Data from the Office of National Health Statistics.

WHERE THE MONEY COMES FROM

Overview

Total national health expenditures, as well as per capita amounts and percentage of distribution by source of funds, for the major sources of funds in selected years from 1960 to 1994 are shown in Table 5.2. As noted above, all the money to pay for health service ultimately comes from the people. Thus, the phrase "where the money comes from" really means "who is collecting the money and how do they do it?"

There are many variants. For example, direct government health care programs (the Department of Veterans Affairs [DVA] hospital system, state mental hospitals, local public general hospitals) are supported mainly by tax revenues. Charitable contributions provide the primary support for the voluntary agencies (e.g., the American Cancer Society). Employer/employee payments are the primary sources of funds for the MCOs.

Private market providers (that is, most physicians and most hospitals) are supported by several sources: direct pay by patients, government tax-supported programs (e.g., Medicaid, a welfare-based system that pays for some health services for the poor [see below]), government social insurance (e.g., Medicare, a part of the Social Security System that pays for some health services for persons aged 65 and over and certain others [also see below]), private insurance (e.g. not-for-profit Blue Cross, or commercial for profit, such as the major life insurance companies), and others.

Figure 5.1 shows that government provided 45% of the health care dollar in 1994, up from about 40% in 1988, and about 22% in 1960 (before the advent of Medicare/Medicaid). In 1994, 32% of the total came from the federal government, the balance from the state and local governments (Levit et al., 1996). Private health insurance, including that provided through MCOs, covered about 33% of payments. Direct out-of-pocket payments accounted for less than 19% of monies paid.

Traditionally, for many patients care has been provided under a direct, private (usually unwritten) contract between themselves and the provider of care. But that care was usually paid for by a "third-party payor" as defined previously, for example, a health insurance company (not for profit or for profit), Medicare, or Medicaid. This picture has been further complicated by the development of managed care. Patient care is still paid for by a third party, but the patient now has a written contract describing in detail what care he/she shall be entitled to, under what circumstances, delivered by whom, in return for the payment made to the

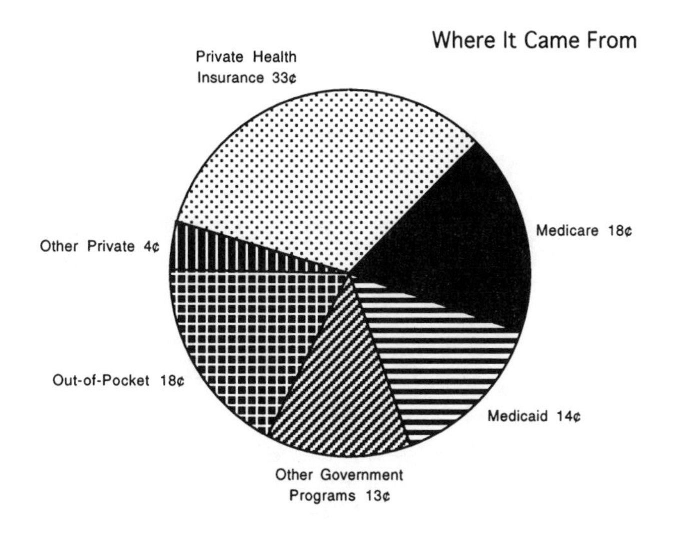

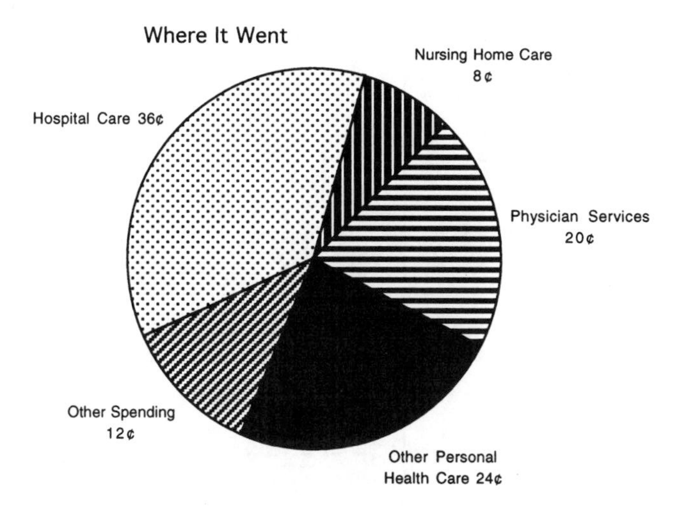

FIGURE 5.1 The nation's health dollar: 1994.

NOTES: Other private includes industrial inplant health services, non-patient revenues, and privately financed construction. Other personal health care includes dental, other professional services, home health care, drugs and other nondurable medical products, vision products and other durable medical products, and other miscellaneous health care services.
Other spending covers program administration and the net cost of private health insurance, government public health, and research and construction.

TABLE 5.2 Personal Health Care Expenditures Aggregate and Per Capita Amounts and Percent Distribution, by Source of Funds: Selected Years 1960–94

			Third-Party Payments							
						Government				
Year	Total	Out-of-Pocket Payments	Total	Private Health Insurance	Other Private Funds	Total	Federal	State and Local	Medicare[1]	Medicaid[2]
					Amount in Billions					
1960	$23.6	$13.1	$10.6	$5.0	$0.4	$5.1	$2.1	$3.0	—	—
1970	63.8	24.9	38.9	14.8	1.6	22.5	14.7	7.8	$7.3	$5.1
1975	114.5	38.1	76.4	28.4	2.7	45.3	30. 9	14.4	15.7	12.9
1980	217.0	60.3	156.8	62.0	7.8	87.0	63.4	23.6	36.4	24.8
1985	376.4	100.6	275.8	113.8	14.1	148.0	111.3	36.7	70.3	39.2
1990	614.7	148.4	466.3	201.8	21.5	243.0	178.1	64.9	109.6	71.7
1991	676.2	155.1	521.1	221.2	23.3	276.6	205.7	70.8	120.2	90.1
1992	739.8	164.4	575.4	242.7	24.3	308.3	234.4	73.9	135.9	102.5
1993	786.5	169.4	617.1	256.4	26.6	334.1	256.8	77.3	148.6	114.1
1994	831.7	174.9	656.8	266.8	28.2	361.8	280.0	81.8	166.1	122.9
					Per Capita Amount					
1960	$124	$69	$56	$26	$2	$27	$11	$16	—	—
1970	297	116	181	69	8	105	68	36	([3])	([3])
1975	510	170	340	126	12	202	138	64	([3])	([3])
1980	923	256	667	264	33	370	270	100	([3])	([3])
1985	1,525	407	1,117	461	57	599	451	149	([3])	([3])
1990	2,369	572	1,797	778	83	936	686	250	([3])	([3])
1991	2,578	591	1,987	843	89	1,054	784	270	([3])	([3])

1992	2,790	620	2,170	916	92	1,163	884	279	([3])	([3])
1993	2,936	632	2,304	957	99	1,247	959	289	([3])	([3])
1994	3,074	646	2,428	986	104	1,337	1,035	302	([3])	([3])
					Percent Distribution					
1960	100.0	55.3	44.7	21.2	1.8	21.7	9.0	12.6	—	—
1970	100.0	39.0	61.0	23.2	2.6	35.3	23.0	12.2	11.4	7.9
1975	100.0	33.3	66.7	24.8	2.4	39.6	27.0	12.5	13.7	11.3
1980	100.0	27.8	72.2	28.6	3.6	40.1	29.2	10.9	16.8	11.4
1985	100.0	26.7	73.3	30.2	3.7	39.3	29.6	9.7	18.7	10.4
1990	100.0	24.1	75.9	32.8	3.5	39.5	29.0	10.6	17.8	11.7
1991	100.0	22.9	77.1	32.7	3.4	40.9	30.4	10.5	17.8	13.3
1992	100.0	22.2	77.8	32.8	3.3	41.7	31.7	10.0	18.4	13.9
1993	100.0	21.5	78.5	32.6	3.4	42.5	32.7	9.8	18.9	14.5
1994	100.0	21.0	79.0	32.1	3.4	43.5	33.7	9.8	20.0	14.8

[1]Subset of Federal funds.
[2]Subset of Federal and State and local funds.
[3]Calculation of per capita estimates is inappropriate.
NOTES: Per capita amounts based on July 1 Social Security area population estimates for each year, 1960–94. Numbers and percents may not add to totals because of rounding.
SOURCE: Health Care Financing Administration, Office of the Actuary: Data from the Office of National Health Statistics.

MCO, usually by the patient's employer. This written contract, with the payor, replaces the old unwritten one with the provider.

Private Health Insurance

About 70% of Americans have some kind of private health insurance coverage (USBoC, 1995), of which there are two kinds (ONCE, 1990). Blue Cross/Blue Shield (BC/BS) has traditionally operated on a not-for-profit basis (although some BC/BS companies were converting to the for-profit mode in the mid-1990s). Any surplus of income over expenditures does not go to share holders. Rather it goes back into the company in the form of expanded services and/or higher salaries for employees.

The commercial companies, for example, the major life insurers such as Metropolitan Life, Travelers, and Aetna, either independently or in partnership with an MCO, operate on a for-profit basis. Some of their surplus of income over expenditures is paid to the owners of the company as profit. The MCOs comprise the most rapidly expanding element of the for-profit sector.

As noted, private health insurance companies took in about one third of all monies collected for health services in 1994. About 85% of this income was paid out for health care provision. The balance went to pay for administrative costs and profits (Levit et al., 1996). About 80% of private health insurance is provided by employers for their workers and their families. It should come as no surprise, therefore, that the services for which the most insurance coverage is available are those used most heavily by the working population. For example, private insurance covered over 34% of hospital costs, 47% of physician services, and 47% of dental services, but only 13% of home care and 3% of nursing home costs (Levit et al., 1996).

Out-of-Pocket Expenditures

Out-of-pocket expenditures include direct payments to providers for non-insured services, extra payments to providers of insurance-covered or managed-care-covered services who bill at an amount higher than the insurance/managed care company pays for that service, and "deductibles" and "coinsurance" on health insurance/managed care benefits (ONCE, 1990; Levit et al., 1996).

A deductible is a flat amount, for example, $200 per individual or $500 per family, that a health care beneficiary must pay out of pocket before insurance coverage begins, for any health services received during some time period (usually a calendar year). Coinsurance is a share, for example

20%, of the payment for each service covered by insurance for which the beneficiary is responsible. In 1994, out-of-pocket payments accounted for about 18% of total expenditures (Figure 5.1).

The "extra charges" mentioned above that some providers levy over what insurance pays are in addition to the coinsurance. Under managed care, beneficiaries receiving health service under the plan from a provider of their choice (a so-called "Point-of-Service" arrangement, see chapter 8) or out of plan entirely will usually pay for some or all of the excess charges out of pocket. Reflecting the different levels of third-party coverage for different health services, whereas out-of-pocket payments accounted for less than 3% of hospital expenditures in 1994, they accounted for over 60% of the costs of medications and "other medical nondurables" (Table 5.3).

Government Spending

Government spending has accounted for an increasing proportion of the health care dollar since 1960. At that time, 5 years before Congress enacted Medicare, government's share was about 22% of the total (Table 5.2). By 1970 it was 35%. It reached 40% in 1980 and has stayed in that range ever since (43.5% in 1994). Government covered close to 60% percent of both hospital and nursing home costs in 1994 (Table 5.3). Together, Medicare and Medicaid covered about 32% of personal health care costs in that year (Figure 5.1).

Medicare

The first U.S. national social insurance program to finance medical care, called Medicare, was established in 1965, created by Title XVIII of the Social Security Act (ONCE, 1990). The legislation was passed by Congress as part of President Lyndon Johnson's "Great Society" program. Originally, it provided payment for some health services for person 65 years of age and older. In 1972 its coverage was broadened to include permanently disabled workers and their dependents who were eligible for old-age, survivors, and disability insurance under Social Security, and persons with end-stage renal disease.

There are two parts to Medicare: hospital insurance (HI), which also covers hospice and home health care, and supplementary medical insurance (SMI), which covers physician services, hospital outpatient care, and certain other services. Medicare HI is funded primarily from Social Security taxes, whereas about two thirds of SMI is funded from general revenues (the balance coming from enrollee premium payments).

TABLE 5.3 National Health Expenditures, by Source of Funds and Type of Expenditure: Selected Calendar Years 1960–94

		Private					Government		
			Consumer						
Year and Type of Expenditure	Total	All Private Funds	Total	Out of Pocket	Private Insurance	Other	Total	Federal	State and Local
1993					Amount in Billions				
National Health Expenditures	$892.3	$505.1	$465.8	$169.4	$296.5	$39.2	$387.2	$278.5	$108.6
Health Services and Supplies	863.1	493.1	465.8	169.4	296.5	27.2	370.0	266.5	103.6
Personal Health Care	786.5	452.3	425.8	169.4	256.4	26.6	334.1	256.8	77.3
Hospital Care	324.2	136.2	123.0	10.0	113.0	13.2	188.0	152.2	35.8
Physician Services	181.1	125.1	122.3	37.0	85.3	2.7	56.0	44.0	12.0
Dental Services	39.2	37.5	37.3	19.1	18.3	0.2	1.7	1.0	0.8
Other Professional Services	46.3	36.0	32.8	18.1	14.7	3.3	10.3	7.4	3.0
Home Health Care	23.0	11.9	8.7	5.6	3.1	3.2	11.1	9.6	1.5
Drugs and Other Medical Non-Durables	75.2	66.0	66.0	46.9	19.1	—	9.2	4.7	4.4
Vision Products and Other Medical Durables	12.6	8.4	8.4	7.5	0.9	—	4.2	4.1	0.1
Nursing Home Care	67.0	28.5	27.3	25.2	2.1	1.2	38.5	24.7	13.8
Other Personal Health Care	17.8	2.8	—	—	—	2.8	15.0	9.2	5.8
Program Administration and Net Cost of Private Health Insurance	51.0	40.7	40.1	—	40.1	0.6	10.3	6.4	3.9
Government Public Health Activities	29.0	25.7	22.4	—	—	—	3.3	3.3	22.4
Research and Construction	29.2	12.0	—	—	—	12.0	17.1	12.1	5.1
Research	14.5	1.2	—	—	—	1.2	13.3	11.2	2.1
Construction	14.7	10.8	—	—	—	10.8	3.9	0.9	2.9

1994									
National Health Expenditures	949.4	528.6	488.1	174.9	313.3	40.4	420.8	303.6	117.2
Health Services and Supplies	919.2	517.1	488.1	174.9	313.3	28.9	402.2	290.3	111.8
Personal Health Care	831.7	469.9	441.6	174.9	266.8	28.2	361.8	280.0	81.8
Hospital Care	338.5	138.9	125.5	9.8	115.7	13.4	199.6	162.7	36.8
Physician Services	189.4	128.5	125.5	35.8	89.6	3.0	60.9	48.6	12.3
Dental Services	42.2	40.4	40.3	20.5	19.8	0.2	1.8	1.0	0.8
Other Professional Services	49.6	38.4	34.7	19.5	15.2	3.7	11.2	8.3	2.9
Home Health Care	26.2	13.0	9.5	6.1	3.4	3.5	13.2	11.4	1.7
Drugs and Other Medical Non-Durables	78.6	68.6	68.6	48.6	20.0	—	10.0	5.2	4.8
Vision Products and Other Medical Durables	13.1	8.6	8.6	7.7	0.9	—	4.5	4.4	0.1
Nursing Home Care	72.3	30.4	29.0	26.8	2.2	1.4	41.8	27.0	14.9
Other Personal Health Care	21.8	3.0	—	—	—	3.0	18.8	11.4	7.4
Program Administration and Net Cost of Private Health Insurance	58.7	47.2	46.5	—	46.5	0.7	11.5	6.6	4.9
Government Public Health Activities	28.8	—	—	—	—	—	28.8	3.7	25.1
Research and Construction	30.2	11.5	—	—	—	11.5	18.7	13.3	5.4
Research	15.9	1.3	—	—	—	1.3	14.7	12.4	2.3
Construction	14.3	10.3	—	—	—	10.3	4.0	0.9	3.1

NOTES: The figure 0.0 denotes less than $50 million. Research and development expenditures of drug companies and other manufacturers and providers of medical equipment and supplies are excluded from research expenditures but are included in the expenditure class in which the product falls. Numbers may not add to totals because of rounding.

SOURCE: Health Care Financing Administration, Office of the Actuary: Data from the Office of National Health Statistics.

Most Medicare beneficiaries use the provider(s) of their choice. Physicians are paid on a fee-for-service basis, according to a fee schedule constructed on the so-called "resource-based relative value system" (RBRVS). (It replaced the old cost-inflation-stimulating "usual and customary fee" system of the mid-1980s.) Hospitals are reimbursed on an episode-of-care basis, the amount of payment for each case determined by a formula based on a fiscal construct called the "Diagnosis-Related Group" (DRG). Managed care was beginning to make its presence felt in the Medicare arena in the mid-1990s (Zarabozo et al., 1996). The long-term outcome of this development is uncertain at this time.

In 1994 total Medicare expenditures were $166.1 billion, covering some of the health care costs for almost 37 million enrollees (Levit et al., 1996). Although about 80% of enrollees incurred some expenditures, about 73% of the total paid for care provided to only 11% of all enrollees. Medicare financed 30% of all spending for hospital care, 20% of physician services costs, and over 36% of home health services costs.

In the mid-1990s, Medicare was in a state of flux. Although the general outlines of the program were likely to remain the same for some time to come, in any given year during the expected life span of this book, things could change. Medicare has always been a political football, no more so than in the period before and during the 1996 Presidential election campaign, when the Democrats claimed that the Republicans were out to "cut Medicare," while the Republicans responded that they were only proposing to reduce the rate of increase in spending for the program and that the Democrats proposed to cut that spending-increase rate too, only less. At the Presidential level, at any rate, the voters bought the Democratic argument.

Over the long haul, however, the health care financing/payment system known as Medicare is in need of rescue/reform. The "babyboomer" population, that extra-large number of people born in the immediate postWorld War II era will reach Medicare eligibility early in the next century, whereas the number of working people available to finance the system through regressive payroll taxes will, in relative terms, be declining.

However, not yet widely recognized in the mid-1990s was the reality that any "permanent rescue" of Medicare required some kind of national health care system covering everyone, with a broad-based financing mechanism for it, to boot. A system such as Medicare, covering through government-based insurance that part of the population requiring the most medical services, but financed narrowly on a payroll rather than a broad-based tax, could not possibly avoid bankruptcy as the need goes up while in relative terms the financing base shrinks. As the fight over the Clinton

Health Plan in 1993–1994 showed (see chapter 9), however, broad-based financing and the regulatory controls that would come with it are something that the U.S. health care industry has historically fought hard to avoid, with almost total success to date.

Medicaid

Along with Medicare, in 1965 Congress also created Medicaid, Title XIX of the Social Security Act (ONCE, 1990). Medicaid is a welfare-based program that provides some coverage for some health services for some of the poor. It is supported by federal and state tax-levy funds and is administered by the states. Each state program is distinct from that of the others. Benefits and who is covered vary widely from state to state. Like Medicare, it generally reimburses providers on a fee-for-service/episode-of-care basis, although in the mid-1990s, managed care was making its presence felt in the Medicaid arena as well.

Title XIX requires a state to provide a set of 21 services in order to be eligible to receive federal funds for their programs, and stipulates that persons eligible for cash payments under the Supplementary Security Income program covering the aged, blind, and disabled, or Aid to Families with Dependent Children (AFDC) (usually referred to as ''Welfare'') be covered by Medicaid. Each state decides who is to be covered by Welfare and what fees are to be paid to providers, however. The 1996 Welfare repeal act will have a major impact on Medicaid, but as of early 1997, the nature of that impact was far from certain.

A combination of low-income eligibility requirements for Welfare, plus low fees paid to providers (many of whom therefore chose not to participate), lead to very limited coverage in many states. On the reverse side of the coin, a few of the wealthier states provided Medicaid coverage for the ''medically indigent.'' These are persons in an income range deemed not to be low enough to qualify them for welfare but low enough to make paying for health services a heavy burden.

Some states, New York for example, had a system whereby the elderly could divest themselves of assets by passing them on to their children, over some period of time. They could thus ''spend down'' to the Medicaid eligibility income and assets levels without losing all of their assets just because the happened to have contracted an illness or negative health condition requiring long-term care. In fact, in 1994, although over two thirds of Medicaid beneficiaries were single mothers and children on AFDC, over two thirds of all expenditures were for the benefit of the aged, the blind, and the disabled (Levit et al., 1996).

In 1988 Medicaid covered about 11% of all personal health care spending. About 23 million people received some kind of Medicaid coverage, but for many, that care was far from comprehensive. Medicaid paid for about 45% of all nursing home care.

Other Government Programs

Among other major government health programs (ONCE, 1990), at the Federal level are the Department of Defense, the Department of Veterans Affairs, and the National Institutes of Health (the federal government's major biomedical research arm); at the state level one finds state public health and mental hospital services; and at the local level there are the local public general hospitals and local public health activities (see also chapter 6).

These government programs are paid for primarily by broad-based tax-levy funds. Together, they consume a relatively small proportion of the national health care budget. For example, in 1994 national expenditures on public health services accounted for less 3% of the total (Table 5.3). By way of comparison, payments for program administration and the net cost of private insurance (administration and profit) together were about 104% higher than expenditures for public health services.

WHERE THE MONEY GOES

Table 5.3 shows the amounts paid for the several major categories of health care and other services as well as the sources of those payments, by type of payor. Spending for personal health services and supplies accounted for about 94% of total national health expenditure in 1994, as previously noted the balance going for government public health activities and research and construction. Personal health care "includes services received by individuals in hospitals, nursing homes, office of physicians, dentists, and other licensed health professionals; home health care; drugs, vision care products, other durable and nondurable medical products;" and that old stand-by "miscellaneous" (ONCE, 1990, p. 4).

In 1994, 37% of all personal health care spending went to hospitals, falling from a peak of 48% in 1982. Hospital payments cover inpatient and outpatient (clinic and emergency room) care costs including such items as capital costs; food; utilities; salaries for administrative, nursing, dietary, maintenance, technology, and other staff; the nonpayroll costs of laboratory and radiology services; physician fees billed through the hospital (e.g., for resident house staff, pathologists and anesthesiologists); and medications.

Along with physicians (both M.D.s and D.O.s) and dentists, there are a number of other categories of health care provider who may be paid directly by the patient or the patient's insurer, for example, psychotherapists (with a Ph.D. or other doctorate, a master's degree, and in some states no degree of any kind), chiropractors, podiatrists (foot care); speech pathologists and audiologists, optometrists (who provide vision testing and eyeglasses) and opticians (who make eyeglasses), and in certain states physical therapists, acupuncturists, naturopaths, homeopaths, and other healers. Payments to them are counted in the "other professional services" category. This category also includes nonhospital outpatient agencies such as kidney dialysis centers, rehabilitation centers, and alcohol and drug treatment centers, as well as the community health centers.

Grouped together under "other spending" are: home health care (preventive, supportive, therapeutic, and rehabilitative); drugs and other medical nondurables (such as bandages); vision products and other medical durables (such hearing aids, braces, and wheel chairs); nursing home care, government public health activities, and the old reliable "all other."

HOW THE MONEY IS PAID OUT

Money is paid for health care by one of five modes: fee-for-service, per unit of care, per episode of care, capitation (which has two meanings), and global budgeting. The predominant mode for paying physicians, dentists, and the private providers in the "other professional services" category above has been fee for service. This piecework system is the oldest form of payment for health services. According to some (Jonas, 1978; Roemer, 1962), it has been a major cause of many problems in the health care delivery system. It should be noted that the majority of people working in the health care delivery system, nurses, administrators, and other institutional staff, as well as some physicians, dentists, and "other health professionals," are paid by salary.

Per unit of care is a method for paying institutions by a unit of time, or a service such as use of the operating room, or the provision of a laboratory test. "Per diem" (by the day) reimbursement for hospital or nursing home care is a common form of per unit of care payment.

Per episode of care is the method used in the DRG system of paying hospitals under Medicare. The hospital receives a flat rate for providing all of the services required to provide complete care for a patient with a given diagnosis. For example, the payment covers bed days, lab tests, X-rays, operations, and so forth, regardless of the actual volume of services used.

The term "capitation" is used in two senses in the health care financing system. A health insurance company or an MCO, contracting with a provider group that may include hospitals in addition to physicians, pays that group a flat rate per enrolled beneficiary (rather than using the traditional item-of-service, "indemnity" payment mechanism). In return the provider group agrees to supply all contract-specified health care services, including hospital, physician, and any other diagnostic-and-treatment services each enrollee might need, during the time period specified in the contract.

The other use of the term "capitation" refers to a method of paying physicians. The physician receives a flat rate for agreeing to provide all medical care to a given patient for a designated period, usually a year. Under managed care this has been increasing at a rapid rate. Until the mid-1990s, this method has been used almost exclusively for primary-care physicians, but the practice is starting to be extended to specialists as well.

Under global budgeting, a health care institution or program receives a lump sum from its sponsoring authority to provide all services to all comers for a given time, usually a year. This is the common way of paying for VA hospitals, state mental hospitals, and local health departments, for example. These institutions in turn may collect reimbursement from various insurance programs, government and private, for patients who have coverage. Monies collected in this manner usually go back to the sponsoring agency to offset the globally budgeted sum.

CONCLUSIONS

The United States spends more on health care services than any other country in the world, both on a gross basis and on a per capita basis. Yet the United States does not have the best health levels in the world when measured, for example, by mortality rate or infant mortality rate (USBoC, 1995). Nor does the United States provide health care coverage for every one of its citizens. As a matter of fact, in 1996, over 40 million Americans had no health care payment coverage of any kind, and it was estimated that at least 29 million more had inadequate coverage (Donelan, et al., 1996).

Although, as noted previously, if one has the right condition, lives in the right place, and has the right health payment coverage, one can indeed get the "best medical care in the world" in the United States, many Americans have diseases or negative health conditions with which the health care delivery system cannot deal effectively, and/or they live in places both urban and rural in which the medical care is inadequate, of less than optimal quality, or simply not available.

At the same, even with the moderating effects of managed care, health care costs continue to increase, if no longer at breathtaking rates, then certainly in breathtaking amounts. A system in which about $25 billion was spent in 1960, accounting for 5.3% of the gross national product will, it is estimated, in current dollars require about $1.5 trillion or 15.9% of the GDP in the year 2,000, and $2.2 trillion or 17.9% of the GDP in 2005 (Burner & Waldo, 1995). And these estimates do not comprehend the implementation of any plan for national health insurance or any other approach to universal coverage.

These facts and figures raise the question ''why?'' both loud and clear. That question cannot be dealt with in any detail here. But as the reader perhaps puts together his or her own answer(s), perhaps the following might be borne in mind. As noted several times, the United States is the only industrialized country that does not have some form of national health insurance or a national health service.

Because it has neither, it has a uniquely complex financing/payment system (as demonstrated by the information in this chapter), requiring enormous amounts of eligibility determination, benefit-checking, co-insurance deductible calculation, billing and collection services, pre-utilization authorization, utilization review, and so forth. Mountains of paperwork and astronomical telephone bills are created, everything costing not only money that could be spent on patient care, but much time as well. Further, as noted, the United States is one of the few industrialized countries that does not have some form of comprehensive health planning system, if not on a national level then at least on a regional one. That lack wastes money too, if in nothing else in the overbuilding of hospital beds in the past (predicted at the time to be overbuilding) with which the system is now very expensively saddled (see chapter 7).

Formerly the country in which physicians on the whole had the highest relative incomes compared with physicians in other countries, the United States is now the only one in which corporate profit-making (through the for-profit MCOs) is a major driver of policy. The United States is the only country in the world in which there is a narrowly financed partial-payment mechanism for the sickest segment of the population (Medicare), a mechanism that encourages the use of the most expensive health care services while ignoring prevention almost completely.

Finally, the United States is the one country that has permitted, indeed encouraged, the development and implementation of the highest levels of ''high-tech'' medicine, without consideration of the moral, ethical, and economic implications of many of those interventions. At the same time, in the U.S. health care system there is widespread, if for the most part unofficial, rationing of health care services by age, gender, race, and economic class (Geiger, 1996; Relman, 1990). At the same time too, health care industry leaders and political figures of many stripes warn that any comprehensive national health insurance system would inevitably ''lead to rationing'' and should thus be avoided.

The explanation for the conundrum set forth in the first three paragraphs of this section is to be found in these facts somewhere. The reader is heartily encouraged to look for it.

REFERENCES

Burner, S. T., & Waldo, D. R. National health expenditure projections, 1994–2005. *Health Care Financing Review, 16,* 221, 1995.

Donelan, K. et al. Whatever happened to the health insurance crisis in the United States? *Journal of the American Medical Association, 276,* 1346, 1996.

Franks, P., & Clancy, C. M. Gatekeeping revisited—Protecting patients from overtreatment. *New England Journal of Medicine, 327,* 427, 1992.

Geiger, H. J. Race and health care—An American dilemma? *New England Journal of Medicine, 335,* 815, 1996.

Jonas, S. *Medical mystery: The training of doctors in the United States*. New York: W. W. Norton, 1978.

Levit, K. R. et al. National health expenditures, 1994. *Health Care Financing Review, 17,* 205, 1996.

ONCE (Office of National Cost Estimates). National health expenditures, 1988. *Health Care Financing Review, 11*(4), 1–54, 1990.

Relman, A. Is rationing inevitable? *New England Journal of Medicine, 322,* 1809, 1990.

Roemer, M. I. On paying the doctor and the implications of different methods. *Journal of Health and Human Behavior, 3*(4), 1962.

USBoC (U.S. Bureau of the Census). *Statistical abstract of the United States: 1990* (110th ed.). Washington, DC: U.S.G.P.O., 1990.

USBoC (U.S. Bureau of the Census). *Statistical abstract of the United States: 1995* (115th ed.). Washington, DC: U.S.G.P.O., 1995.

Zarabozo, C. et al. Medicaid managed care: Numbers and trends. *Health Care Financing Review, 17,* 243, 1966.

Chapter 6
Government

As we noted in chapter 1, the U.S. government operates neither the health care delivery system nor the health services financing system in anything close to the entirety of either. In fact, in the United States the government is less involved with the provision of health care than it is in any other industrialized country in the world. Perhaps the most important reason for this difference is the strength of the private medical, hospital, insurance company, and now managed care sectors of the health services economy and their opposition to what they term ''government control and interference'' (except of course in certain select areas that are not profitable or are technically difficult to deal with, such as care of the sick poor, care of the mentally ill, providing payment for both short- and long-term care of the elderly, and infectious disease control). Restricted as the government's role is compared with that in other nations, however, in terms of dollars spent (see chapter 5) it still looms rather large, and thus deserves our attention.

SOME HISTORY

The health care role that government does have in the United States has developed and expanded gradually over a long period of time. In his Preface to a seminal book of the 1940s by Bernhard J. Stern, W. G. Smillie, one of the first medical sociologists and a noted public health authority of the day, said (Stern, 1946, p. xiii):

> Our forefathers certainly had no concept of responsibility of the Federal Government, nor of the state government, for health protection of the people. This was solely a local governmental responsibility. When Benjamin Franklin wrote ''Health is Wealth'' in the Farmers' Almanac, he was

> saying that health was a commodity to be bought, to be sold, to be conserved, or to be wasted. But he considered that health conservation was the responsibility of the individual, not of government. The local community was responsible only for the protection of its citizens against the hazards of community life.
>
> Thus government responsibility for health protection consisted of (a) promotion of sanitation and (b) communicable disease control. The Federal Constitution, as well as the Constitutions of most of the states, contains no reference or intimation of a federal or state function in medical care. The care of the sick poor was a local community responsibility from earliest pioneer days. This activity was assumed first by voluntary philanthropy; later, it was transferred, and became an official governmental obligation.

Professor Stern continued that line of thinking in his own introduction to his book (1946, pp. 4–5):

> Government action in the field has traditionally been limited to the care of the indigent and has been dominated in its scope and administration by the restraining influences of the parochial poor laws. Gradually, and especially after the passage of the Social Security Act and during [World War II], government medical care has increasingly been furnished to some nonindigent groups. New patterns of government medical care are being formulated and the role of local, state, and federal governments in the field is changing. . . . The attitudes of the medical profession and of the public toward government medical programs will determine whether these resources are to be used progressively to distribute more medical care of higher quality to the American people.

What a contemporary ring this last sentence has, written as it was about 50 years prior to the writing of this book (see also chapter 9).

Even without any kind of national health system, however, government at all jurisdictional levels in the United States is much more heavily involved in the health care delivery system in both degree and kind in 1996 than it was in 1946. Consider, for example, such initiatives as Medicare and Medicaid, new regulatory powers, and support of biomedical research and health professions education. But certain characteristics have remained unchanged. They are most significant. To quote Smillie again (Stern, 1946, p. xiv):

> Practically all governmental procedures in medical care stem from the original local community responsibility for the care of the sick poor, and many of our great municipal hospitals, clinics, and health services of today still bear the stigma of pauperism.

The pauper stigma, signifying that ''poor equals bad'' and that poverty is the fault of the poor, is still attached to much government activity in direct care delivery (although certain health department services have managed to escape the taint). It is rooted in the Protestant ethic, which held people directly accountable for their state in life. The legal implementation of the Protestant ethic goes back at least as far as the Elizabethan Poor Laws in England (de Schweinitz, 1943/1961).

Although in our society today some may accept socioeconomic explanations as to why some people are well off and others are destitute, the attitudes of many toward the proper role of government in health care are still colored by old values and prejudices toward the poor and people of color (Jonas, 1986). And the health status of the latter groups is different from that of the nation as a whole. For example, one study reported in 1996 (Geronimus et al., 1996, p. 1552) that:

> When they were compared with the nationwide age-standardized annual death rates for whites, the death rates for both sexes in each of the [studied] poverty areas were excessive, especially among blacks. . . . Boys in Harlem [a predominately black district in New York City] who reached the age of 15 had a *37 percent* chance of surviving to the age of 65; for girls the likelihood was *65 percent* [emphasis added].

And some wonder just why it is that some young Black men seem to hold themselves to a different standard of behavior than that considered standard for the society as a whole.

Many questions remain about the role of government in health today, some of which have resonated for decades. In his Preface to the landmark report of the Institute of Medicine's Committee on The Future of Public Health, Dr. Richard Remington summarized them well (IOM, 1988, pp. v–vi):

> But what is the most appropriate nature of that governmental presence? How should government's role relate to that of the private sector? How should governmental responsibility for public health be apportioned among local, state, and federal levels? Should government be the health care provider of last resort or does it have a greater responsibility? Should public health consist only of a necessary residuum of activities not met by private providers? How should governmental activities directed toward the maintenance of an environment conducive to health be apportioned among various agencies? But above all, just what is public health? What does it include and what does it exclude? Based on an appropriate definition, what kinds of programs and agencies should be constructed to meet the needs and demands of the public, which is often resistant to an increasing role, or at least an increasing cost, of government?

In the mid-1990s, the questions had yet to be answered. The public debate about the role of government in health care had sharply diminished in intensity following the defeat of the Clinton Health Plan (see chapter 9), however, even though a very significant role for government in health care delivery is justified by the amount of money government spends on it alone. That role has a Constitutional basis as well.

THE CONSTITUTIONAL BASIS OF GOVERNMENT AUTHORITY IN HEALTH CARE

To understand government operations in the health care delivery system, it is essential to understand the structure of the government itself.[1] A basic principle of the United States Constitution is that sovereign power is to be shared between the federal and state governments, a principle called federalism. At its heart, the United States Constitution is an agreement between the original 13 states to delegate some of their inherent powers to the federal government. As part of this agreement, in the Tenth Amendment to the Constitution, the states (and through them the people at large) explicitly reserved to themselves the rest of the power: "The powers not delegated to the United States by the Constitution, nor prohibited by it to the states, are reserved to the states respectively, or to the people." Because it is not explicitly mentioned in the Constitution, among the powers reserved to the states is the police power. It is the latter which forms the basis of the states' role in health (Mustard, 1945). As Grad points out (1990, p. 10):

> In the states, government authority to regulate for the protection of public health and to provide health services is based on the "police power"—that is, the power to provide for the health, safety, and welfare of the people. It is not necessary that this power be expressly stated, because it is a plenary power that every sovereign government has, simply by virtue of being a sovereign government. For purposes of the police power, the state governments—which antedate the federal government—are sovereign governments. . . . The exercise of the police power is really what government is about. It defines government.

[1]The *Public health law manual* by Frank P. Grad (1990), *Health and the law* by Tom Christoffel (1982), and "The legal basis for public health" by E. P. Richards and K. C. Rathbun, in Scutchfield and Keck's *Principles of public health practice* (1996) are valuable guides to the legal basis of government activity in health care and to the many legal procedures involved in the enforcement of public health law.

Among the states' other inherent powers are those of delegation of their own authority. The states have used this to create a third tier of government, local government. Most states have delegated some of their health powers to that tier. The Constitutional basis of the federal government's health authority is found in the powers to tax and spend to provide for the general welfare, and to regulate interstate and foreign commerce (see the Preamble and Article I, Section 8 of the Constitution) (Grad, 1990).

The other basic Constitutional principle affecting health and health services is "separation of powers." The Constitution divides the sovereign power of the federal government among three branches of government: executive, legislative, and judicial. Under separation of powers, each branch of the federal government has its own authority and responsibility, spelled out in the Constitution. Further, the Constitution spells out curbs on the powers of each branch, exercised by the other two. This arrangement is called the system of checks and balances.

(One very important check on the power of both the federal legislative and executive branches, judicial review of the Constitutionality of their actions, is not found in the Constitution, however. It was established early in the 19th century by the third Chief Justice of the Supreme Court, John Marshall, and his colleagues on the bench. It has become an accepted part of the United States Constitutional system only because the other two branches have granted the Court that authority in practice and have followed its determinations.)

The state governments followed fairly closely the tripartite form of government, with checks and balances (and the 14th Amendment extended federal judicial review to certain state government actions as well). At the local level, the boundaries between branches at times become blurred, however. For example, in some suburban and rural areas the local chief executive officer presides over the local legislative body. Nevertheless, in most United States jurisdictions, separation of powers is a major principle of government.

THE HEALTH CARE FUNCTIONS OF GOVERNMENT

The Legislative Branch

At each level of government, federal, state, and local, each of the three branches of government has responsibility and authority for health and health services. Legislatures create the laws that establish the means to safeguard the public's health, in matters ranging from the assurance of a pure water supply to protecting the health of workers in their places of employment. The legislatures enact the legal framework within which the health care delivery system functions, deciding which individuals and institutions are authorized to deliver what services to which persons under what conditions and requirements.

Legislatures may impose certain requirements for planning and development of the system (see chapter 7). If the government is to participate in health care financing (see chapter 5), or directly deliver services (see this chapter and chapter 3) or support research efforts, the legislature must first establish the legal authority for those programs.

The Judiciary

The judicial branches at the three levels of government have important powers relating to health and health services. They cannot apprehend transgressors, or prosecute them, or carry out punishment on their own, however. Thus they must work in concert with the law enforcement arms of the executive branches, under the authority granted to them by their respective legislatures. Together, the judicial and executive branches form the civil and criminal justice systems.

The judiciary supports the work of the other branches of government. For example, although it is a state legislature that creates the licensing law for physicians and the executive branch that administers it, it is the judicial system that determines the guilt or innocence of a person charged with practicing medicine without a license. The judicial system handles civil disputes arising from the provision of health services, for example, through the process of malpractice litigation. It protects the rights of individuals under the due process and equal protection clauses of the Fifth and Fourteenth Amendments to the Constitution. The criminal justice system also plays a vital role in safeguarding the public's health. For example, it enforces sanitary protection and pollution control legislation, with criminal sanctions if necessary.

The Executive Branch

In common parlance, the term "government in health care" refers to the executive branch that delivers health care services, drafts and enforces provider/payor regulations, and administers financing programs, not the legislature that creates the programs or regulatory authority, or the courts that settle disputes arising from them and adjudicate violations of them. As it does in common parlance, in the remainder of this chapter the term "government" refers to the executive branch of government.

Provision of Personal Health Services

At the federal level, personal health services are provided for the most part to *categories* of person: members of the uniformed services and their families, Native Americans, and veterans, for example. State governments provide personal health services for the most part to persons who have specific diseases, such as mental illness and tuberculosis. Local government's personal health services generally are for the poor. There are occasional overlaps. For example, governments at all levels provide health services for prisoners, one category of person.

Provision of Community Health Services

Government at all levels is the major provider of the traditional ''public health'' services, such as pure water supply and sanitary sewage disposal, food and drug inspection and regulation, communicable disease control (e.g., immunization, and the control of sexually transmitted diseases), vital statistics, and public health laboratory work.

Certain community health activities are shared with the private sector. For example, in public health education, voluntary agencies such as the American Cancer Society and the American Heart Association are important participants. Private refuse companies do much of the solid waste collection. Private organizations like the Sierra Club and the Natural Resources Defense Council are active in environmental protection. Private institutions also play a vital role in health sciences education and research.

Health Services Financing

As described in chapter 5, Government participates in the financing system in three ways. First, it pays for the operation of its own programs, both personal and community. It does this directly, for example, as in the federal government's veterans hospital system or a municipal hospital serving primarily the poor. It also does this indirectly, for example, as in the federal government's provision of grants to state governments to help provide care in state mental hospitals, and to help operate the state's public health agencies. The states in turn indirectly support local government public health activities by providing money for that purpose.

Second, through grants and contracts to nongovernmental agencies (and in certain cases, other governmental agencies) governments support other types of health-related programs, for example, in biomedical research and medical education. Third, and this is by far and away their major role in financing, under such programs as Medicare and Medicaid governments pay providers for the delivery of care to third parties. As noted in chapter

5, federal, state, and local public funds accounted for about 45% of national health expenditures in 1994, up from 42% in 1988.

THE FEDERAL GOVERNMENT AND THE PROVISION OF HEALTH SERVICES

Many federal agencies are involved in the delivery of personal and community health services (Brandt, 1996). The U.S. Department of Health and Human Services (USDHHS) is the most important federal actor in health care. Including its social-service functions, in the mid-1990s the Department operated about 250 different programs (USDHHS, 1996). These are two other federal agencies with major health services responsibilities: the Departments of Veterans Affairs and Defense. Other federal agencies with significant health-related responsibilities include the Department of Agriculture (nutrition policy, meat and poultry inspection, food stamps), the Environmental Protection Agency, and the Department of Labor (administering the Occupational Safety and Health Act).

USDHHS

The Mission of the USDHHS is to (USDHHS, 1996):

> [P]rotect and promote the health, social and economic well-being of all Americans and in particular those least able to help themselves—children, the elderly, persons with disabilities, and the disadvantaged—by helping them and their families develop and maintain healthy, productive, and independent lives. [p. 1]

The USDHHS has 10 major operating divisions. (Until March 31, 1995, that number was 11. On April 1, 1995 [no foolin'] the Social Security Administration became an independent agency.) Eight of the 10 USDHHS divisions are concerned with health. They are the seven grouped under what is officially known as the United States Public Health Service (USPHS), plus the Health Care Financing Administration, which administers the Medicare and Medicaid programs at the federal level.

As of 1996 the Public Health Service existed in name only. No longer was it an operating administrative entity. The position of Assistant Secretary for Health, the person who had formerly administered the USPHS as a single agency, was abolished. The directors of each of its former constituents, described briefly below, were left to report directly to the

Secretary of Health and Human Services (McGinnis, 1996). It remained to be seen for how long this cumbersome system would exist.

Public Health Service

The Public Health Service had a long and proud history, dating to a 1798 act creating the Marine Hospital Service (MHS) (Mustard, 1945; Schmeckebier, 1975; Stern, 1946). In 1878 Congress added foreign quarantine responsibilities to the work of the MHS. This led in 1889 to the development of a quasi-military personnel system (the "Commissioned Corps" of the PHS). The Corps was made up largely of career medical people, commanded (symbolically in recent years) by the Surgeon General of the United States.

The PHS continued to gain responsibilities over time. Following the end of World War II it grew rapidly, with: the passage of the Hospital Survey and Construction (Hill–Burton) Act of 1946; the major expansion of the National Institutes of Health; the creation of the Communicable Disease Center in Atlanta (now the Centers for Disease Control and Prevention); and the development of drug abuse control, mental retardation, and mental health centers, and comprehensive health planning activities, among others.

As of 1996, the seven former USPHS divisions were (USDHHS, 1996): the Health Resources and Services Administration, the Centers for Disease Control and Prevention, the Food and Drug Administration, the National Institutes of Health, the Substance Abuse and Mental Health Services Administration, the Indian Health Service, and the Agency for Health Care Policy and Research. Collectively these agencies carry out a wide variety of functions: regulating, providing direct personal and community health services, providing financial support for a variety of health services through grants and contracts, direct research, and providing the principal federal support of biomedical research in nongovernment agencies.

The *Health Resources and Services Administration* (HRSA, 1996) runs the direct service programs of DHHS for "medically needy" persons, primarily through community and migrant health centers; supports efforts to improve the education and use of the nation's health personnel; supports efforts to improve health care delivery programs, especially for underserved populations; attempts to improve the use of health facilities; aids in increasing the number of minorities in the health professions; administers the National Health Service Corps (which provides financial aid to selected medical students in return for a service commitment from them for work in underserved communities upon the completion of their training); and participates in the acquired immunodeficiency syndrome (AIDS) control program in a variety of ways.

The *Centers for Disease Control and Prevention* (CDCP) is the national public health agency primarily responsible for prevention efforts. Its programs are aimed at preventing and controlling disease and personal injury, directing foreign and interstate quarantine operations, developing programs for health education and health promotion, improving the performance of clinical laboratories, and developing the standards necessary to insure safe and healthful working conditions for all working people. Through the National Center for Health Statistics, the CDCP collects and publishes a wide variety of vital, health, and health services data. It maintains the nation's reference laboratories and supports laboratory training programs. It also awards project grants to state and local health agencies to support immunization, particularly for children.

The task of the *Food and Drug Administration* (FDA) is to protect the public against food, drug, and medical devices product hazards, and to assure drug potency and effectiveness. Thus, the FDA regulates prescription drugs and over-the-counter medications, biological products, and human blood and its derivatives. The focus is on the assurance of the efficacy and safety of a product before marketing, and on the assurance of continuing quality after approval. Medical devices are regulated in a similar manner. Radiological equipment is also regulated, the goal being to control radiation exposure to the public. In addition, the FDA has responsibilities in veterinary medicine and toxicology.

The regulatory programs of the FDA, especially those focusing on the efficacy and safety of drugs and medical devices, are sometimes controversial. Industry spokespeople state that the entry of useful drugs to the market is at times unnecessarily delayed by a lengthy and expensive approval process. Supporters of that process recall, for example, the thalidomide disaster. Nevertheless, in the mid-1990s the FDA did manage to introduce internal reforms significantly speeding up the drug-review process (MacPherson, 1996).

In 1996 the FDA brought intense right-wing opprobrium on itself (AHA, 1996; Weyrich, 1996) by proposing to regulate tobacco products as drug-delivery devices (Kessler et al., 1996). The proposed policy was based on the correct understanding that adult cigarette smoking almost invariably begins in childhood and that the development and enforcement of a series of regulations designed to significantly reduce youth cigarette smoking could have a major impact on the health of the nation over a period of time.

Through its multiple institutes, such as the National Cancer Institute and the National Heart, Lung, and Blood Institute, the *National Institutes of Health* (NIH) is responsible for supporting and carrying out biomedical research. Its primary mission focuses on basic biomedical research at the organ system, tissue, cellular, and subcellular level. Although other federal agencies also support biomedical research, as of 1990 the NIH alone accounted for about two thirds of the federal investment in it. NIH has its own (intramural) research program on its campus in Bethesda, Maryland and provides funds for research at many other institutions around the country through (extramural) grants and contracts. NIH also fosters research by supporting training, resource development, and construction.

The *Substance Abuse and Mental Health Services Administration* (SAMHSA) supports treatment services for illicit drug and alcohol abuse; conducts clinical and biomedical research in its own laboratories; helps the states provide mental health services; funds extramural research, research training, and prevention programs through grants and contracts; monitors substance abuse and supports innovative treatment-and-prevention projects nationwide.

The *Indian Health Service* provides health care for about 1,400,000 Native Americans and Alaska Natives who live on or near Indian reservations. Health services provided include hospital, ambulatory, preventive, and rehabilitative care, and community sanitation. The Indian Health Service has a system of about 40 hospitals and more than 100 other health facilities in 27 states, and a network of providers working on contract.

The *Agency for Health Care Policy and Research* "supports crosscutting research on health care systems, health care costs, and effectiveness of medical treatments" (USDHHS, 1996, p. 1).

Office of Disease Prevention and Health Promotion

This is another important federal health agency that was reorganized out of existence in 1995. Its primary responsibility was to strengthen the health-promotion and disease-prevention activities of DHHS in collaboration with the PHS and other DHHS agencies. In 1989 it published *The Guide to Clinical Preventive Services* (USPSTF, 1989), the product of the work of the United States Preventive Services Task Force. Over a 3-year period, that body reviewed and evaluated about 170 different clinical preventive interventions in common use.

In 1990 ODPHP (Office of Disease Prevention and Health Promotion) published *Healthy People 2000: National Health Promotion and Disease Prevention Objectives* (USDHHS, 1990), a set of goals and specific health objectives to be achieved by the nation as a whole by the year 2000, in 22 priority areas ranging from exercise to cancer prevention, from environmental health to immunization, for the health care delivery system and our people as a whole. A follow-up work, *Healthy People 2000: Midcourse Review and 1995 Revisions* was published in 1995 (USPHS, 1995).

Other Federal Departments

Many other federal departments have some health responsibilities, as previously noted. Several are discussed here.

The *Department of Veterans Affairs* (DVA) provides many services to veterans. After military service, the United States veteran becomes entitled to a remarkably broad range of health services, through a health care subsystem the precise equivalent of which is not found in any other nation in the world. This fact is doubtless related to the lack of a national health insurance program for the general population and the political power of the veterans' organizations.

A veteran is defined as anyone who served 90 days or more in an armed service, but a veteran must have received an honorable or general discharge in order to be automatically eligible. Thus, for eligibility there is a "moral means test" based on discharge status.

Among those veterans holding honorable or general discharges, there are four overlapping groups eligible to receive DVA medical care: (1) those with service-connected disabilities or certain other qualifying characteristics such as having been exposed to herbicides in Vietnam; (2) recipients of DVA pensions; (3) veterans 65 years and older; (4) those meeting certain income means tests (DVA, 1990). By 1995, only 12% of patients treated in VA hospitals had service-connected disabilities (GAO, 1996). Thus veterans other than those in categories 1 and 2 may have to pay a portion of the charges for their care.

The DVA owns the largest centrally directed hospital and clinic system in the United States. In 1995 the DVA was operating 173 medical centers providing about 14.7 million hospital days of care (GAO, 1996). This number was down sharply from the 26 million hospital days of care provided in 1980. In addition to the medical centers, there were 376 outpatient clinics, 136 nursing homes, and 39 "domiciliaries." Reflecting the national trend toward moving certain kinds of treatment and care out of the hospital, there were altogether about 26.5 outpatient visits, up from 15.2 million in 1980. In 1995 the DVA's annual health care budget was over $16.2 billion.

In the mid-1990s, a major challenge facing the health care delivery system of the DVA was the rapid aging of the veteran population, these are parents of the "baby boomers" who will themselves be weighing down the Social Security/Medicare system during the first third of the next century. In response to this and other challenges, reflecting the numbers cited just above, as John Igelhart noted (1996, p. 140):

> The department is decentralizing, reducing its inpatient capacity, reallocating resources to ambulatory care, and simplifying the convoluted method

> Congress designed to determine which veterans are eligible to receive medical services. These changes, which are shaking the rigid foundations of the Veterans Affairs system . . . represent, in many respects, an attempt to transform the department's vast medical system along the lines of managed care.

The Department of Defense (DOD) oversees the health services of the various branches of the military. Each of the armed forces, the Army, Navy, Air Force, and Marines, has its own network of health facilities hospitals, clinics, and field posts (ASD, 1990, 1996). All DOD health personnel are members of the military, salaried according to their military ranks (without relation to the specific services they render). The same basic structure prevails in times of war or peace. Health promotion and disease prevention are emphasized and integrated with the delivery of treatment services.

Through both its own facilities and contracting arrangements with civilian providers, DOD provides health services to members of the armed forces, their dependents, surviving dependents of servicepeople killed while on active duty, and military retirees and their dependents. Servicemen and women are eligible for retirement benefits after a minimum of 20 years of service. The health services part of that package is paid in addition to the DVA benefits for which they may be eligible.

An unusual aspect of military medical departments is that they are charged not only with providing a full range of direct health services but also with providing for the environmental health and protection of their military communities. This unification of administrative responsibility for personal and community preventive and treatment services is rarely found elsewhere in the United States health care delivery system.

The U.S. Department of Agriculture (USDA) provides some health services for agricultural families and farm workers, control programs for animal diseases, and plant health services. The USDA also operates nutrition services, such as the Women and Infants Care (WIC) program, school breakfast and lunch programs, and the Food Stamp program, which helps poor people to buy food. It conducts research on the nutrient composition of foods, food consumption, and nutritional requirements. In cooperation with the USDHHS, it periodically issues dietary guidelines for the nation. It supervises food-safety regulations in cooperation with the FDA, and grades meats and other foods for consumers. It also has programs in nutrition education and research.

Focusing on preventive activities in the workplace, the *Occupational Safety and Health Administration (OSHA)* is part of the Department of Labor. OSHA uses criteria developed by the National Institute of Occupational Safety and Health (NIOSH), part of the CDCP, to set national standards for occupational safety and health (Brock & Tyson, 1985). The major responsibilities of OSHA are to develop workplace health and safety standards, to enforce and gain compliance with the standards, to engage in education and training, to help the states in occupational safety and health matters, and to aid business in meeting OSHA requirements. There are a few industries that are not covered by OSHA. For example, the health and safety of miners is the province of the Bureau of Mines in the Department of the Interior.

The *Environmental Protection Agency (EPA)* is an independent (nondepartmental) agency (elevated to cabinet-level status during the Clinton Administration) that has major responsibilities for the control of air and water quality and pollution, solid-waste disposal, pesticide contamination, radiation hazards, and toxic substances (EPA, 1988, 1989). The EPA conducts research on air, water, and land pollution-control technology and the effects of pollution on humans, develops criteria and issues national standards for pollutants, and enforces compliance with these standards.

THE STATE GOVERNMENTS' ROLE IN HEALTH SERVICES[2]

Introduction

As at the federal level, at the state level many different agencies are involved in health services. For example, in most states departments other than the health department provide two of the important health-related functions managed primarily by the states: mental illness treatment services (by the department of mental health or its equivalent) and Medicaid operations (by the welfare department or its equivalent). Furthermore, the licensing authority for health personnel sometimes resides in the education department, vocational rehabilitation is often found in a special agency, occupational health in the labor department, environmental protection in a separate department, and school health with local boards of education. Most states also have a board of health, usually appointed by the governor, which has varying administrative, policy, and advisory functions.

In the 1920s, political struggles with the private practitioners (referred to in chapter 3) led to a limitation of service responsibilities for both the state and local health departments. Haven Emerson, a leading public health

[2]A comprehensive review of state and local (as well as federal) public health activities, with an extensive bibliography, is to be found in Appendix A of *The future of public health* (IOM, 1988). See also *Public health agencies 1991* (PHF, 1991), as of 1996 the most recent edition of this report.

official of the time, defined the ''Basic Six'' services appropriate for departments of public health. They were: vital statistics, public health laboratories, communicable disease control, environmental sanitation, maternal and child health, and public health education (Wilson & Neuhauser, 1976, p. 204).

The Association of State and Territorial Health Officials (ASTHO) has defined a state health program as

> A set of identifiable services organized to solve health related problems or to meet specific health or health related needs, provided to or on behalf of the public, by or under the direction of an organizational entity in a State Health Agency [SHA], and for which reasonably accurate estimates of expenditures can be made. (ASTHO, 1980, p. vii)

Using this definition, ASTHO identified six program areas for SHAs: ''personal health, environmental health, health resources, laboratory, general administration and services, and funds to local health departments not allocated to program areas'' (ASTHO, 1980, p. 9). Although the number is still six, in some states the content of the work has expanded well beyond that comprehended by the ''Basic Six'' (Dandoy, 1996).

Since World War II, as the health care delivery system has become vastly more complex, there have been an increasing number of public health and health services interests requiring protection. In response, governments have vastly expanded the responsibilities of both state and local departments of health and other health-related governmental agencies. Those responsibilities now include, for example, regulation and quality assurance for physicians, hospitals, and other provider/payor agencies, including institutional licensure, planning (what there is of it), and ever-more complex environmental protection functions. And, as noted above, state and local health-related activities outside of the health departments have expanded as well.

Health Statistics

Among the oldest of public health functions is the collection and analysis of vital and health statistics. Data on births, deaths, marriages, and divorces, and incidence of the several reportable (primarily infectious) diseases are collected by the local health authorities and forwarded to the state level. There they are codified and analyzed, often by various demographic characteristics such as age, gender, marital status, ethnicity, and geographic location. Each state then forwards its collected data to the National Center for Health Statistics of the Centers for Disease Control and Prevention for further analysis and publication.

Licensing

Licensing is a basic government function in health care. The licensing process for individual practitioners first establishes minimum standards for qualification. It then applies those standards to applicants to determine who may and who may not deliver what kinds of health services. Licensing of health care institutions sets minimum standards for the facility and its personnel as a group, applies the standards, and determines whether the institution may operate.

The licensing authority is one of the most significant of the health powers residing with the states. The manner in which it is used is a major determinant of the character of the United States' health care delivery system. The medical licensing system is particularly significant in that regard. Because no one can practice medicine without a license, the system has given physicians tight control over the central product of the health care delivery system—medical services.

By exercising this control, physicians have largely determined the structure of the health care delivery system: how it is organized, the types and functions of the institutions, and the powers of the several categories of personnel who work in it. As we have seen on more than one occasion throughout this book, however, despite the provisions of the licensing laws, that physician authority is being challenged by the MCOs.

THE LOCAL GOVERNMENTS' ROLE IN HEALTH SERVICES

A local health department (LHD) is a unit of either state or local government focusing exclusively on a ''substate'' geographic area, usually a well-defined one considered by virtually any observer to be ''local'' in nature—a county, city, town, parish, or village. In the mid-1990s, there were about 2,900 local health departments throughout the United States, employing about 192,000 people, of whom 145,000 were full-time workers, providing health services of one kind or another to about 40 million people at any annual cost of about $8 billion (Rawding & Wasserman, 1996).

The activities of most LHDs are limited for the most part to some version of the Basic Six, although in recent years some have also become involved in the direct delivery of ambulatory services to the poor. Following the state and federal models, certain local health services are provided by various agencies other than health departments. For example, cities and counties are likely to place their hospitals for the poor, their mental health services and environmental protection including water supply, sanitary sewage disposal, and solid waste disposal under separate agencies.

Commonly, LHDs provide one or more of the following services: immunization, environmental surveillance, tuberculosis control, maternal and child health, school health, venereal disease control, chronic disease control, home care, family planning, ambulatory care, and health code enforcement. Thus, the LHDs, in cooperation with SHAs and other state agencies, particularly in environmental health, are the backbone of the system for providing public health and preventive services to the people.

PROBLEMS IN PUBLIC HEALTH

State and local public health services, and indeed federal ones too, face many problems. The state of affairs as of the mid-1990s was still best summarized by the Committee on the Future of Public Health which published its report in 1988 (IOM, 1988, pp. 1–2):

> Many of the major improvements in the health of the American people have been accomplished through public health measures. . . . But the public has come to take the success of public health for granted. . . . [T]his nation has lost sight of its public health goals and has allowed the system of public health activities to fall into disarray.
>
> Public health is what we, as a society, do collectively to assure the conditions in which people can be healthy. . . . [M]any problems demonstrate the need to protect the nation's health through effective, organized, and sustained effort by the public sector. . . . The current state of our abilities for effective public health action . . . is cause for national concern. . . . [W]e have slackened our public health vigilance nationally, and the health of the public is unnecessarily threatened as a result. . . .
>
> Successes as great as those of the past are still possible, but not without public concern and concerted action to restore America's public health capacity. This volume envisions the future of public health, analyzes the current situation and how it developed, and presents a plan of action that will, in the committee's judgement, provide a solid foundation for a strong public health capability throughout the nation.

The Committee's report is recommended to those readers who are concerned with the future of public health in the United States.

CONCLUSIONS

Although as we have seen, government is heavily involved in health and health care in the United States, United States politics and the United

States economic system significantly limit the degree of that involvement. Government provides the legal underpinning for the system through the licensing laws. It regulates the financial workings of the system and its quality of care. Government is also a direct financier and a direct provider of service. It is preeminent in community health services and plays an important part in supporting health sciences education and research.

The resistance to "government interference in the practice of medicine" is still very prominent among private medical practitioners, however. And they have been joined in that regard by the powerful interests of the for-profit managed care sector (see chapter 8). In many laws concerning the health care delivery system (for example, the Social Security amendments establishing the Medicare program) such interference is expressly prohibited.

Most providers of both the individual and corporate variety (often grudgingly) recognize the reality that government is already heavily involved in the practice of medicine. As noted, they welcome participation in certain critical areas: licensing; care of the mentally ill, the tubercular, and the poor; and community health services. But it is likely that the questions about the proper role of government in health for our country today, summarized so well by Dr. Remington at the beginning of this chapter, cannot be fruitfully resolved until the place and the power of the private health services provider sector in the health care delivery system as a whole is redefined.

REFERENCES

AHA (American Hospital Association). Currents: Ethics. *Hospitals and Health Networks*, September 5, 1996, p. 12.

ASD (Assistant Secretary of Defense for Health Affairs). *Report on the reorganization of military health care*. Washington, DC: U.S.G.P.O., June 1990.

ASD (Assistant Secretary of Defense [Health Affairs]). Office of the Assistant Secretary for Health Affairs. Washington, DC: U.S.G.P.O., 1996.

ASTHO (Association of State and Territorial Health Officials). *Comprehensive national public health programs, of state and territorial health agencies, fiscal year 1978*. Silver Springs, MD: Author, 1980.

Brandt, E. The federal contribution to public health. In F. D. Scutchfield & C. W. Keck (Eds.), *Principles of public health practice*. Albany, NY: Delmar, 1996.

Brock, W. E., & Tyson, P. R. *All about OSHA*. Washington, DC: U.S.G.P.O., 1985.

Christoffel, T. *Health and the law*. New York: Free Press, 1982.

Comptroller General. *Military medicine is in trouble.* Washington, DC: U.S.G.P.O., 1979.

Dandoy, S. The state public health department. In F. D. Scutchfield & C. W. Keck (Eds.), *Principles of public health practice.* Albany, NY: Delmar, 1996.

de Schweinitz, K. *England's road to social security.* New York: A. S. Barnes, 1961. (Original work published 1943.)

DVA (Department of Veterans' Affairs). *Federal benefits for veterans and dependents.* Washington, DC: U.S.G.P.O., January 1990.

EPA (Environmental Protection Agency). *Environmental progress and challenges: EPA's update.* Washington, DC: U.S.G.P.O., 1988.

EPA. (*Your guide to the United States environmental protection agency.* Washington, DC: EPA Office of Public Affairs, 1989.

GAO (General Accounting Office). *VA health care: Opportunities for service delivery efficiencies within existing resources.* GAO/HEHS-96-121, Washington, DC: Author, July 1996.

Geronimus, A. T. et al. Excess mortality among blacks and whites in the United States. *New England Journal of Medicine, 335,* 1552, 1996.

Grad, F. *The public health law manual* (2nd ed.). Washington, DC: American Public Health Association, 1990.

Hayward, R. R. et al. Inequities in health services among insured Americans. *New England Journal of Medicine, 318,* 1507, 1988.

HRSA (Health Resources and Services Administration). *Profile.* Washington, DC, USDHHS, 1996.

Igelhart, J. K. Reform of the Veterans Affairs health care system. *New England Journal of Medicine, 335,* 1407, 1996.

IOM (Institute of Medicine). *The future of public health.* Washington, DC: Author, 1988.

Jonas, S. On homelessness and the American way. *American Journal of Public Health, 76,* 1084, 1986.

Kessler, D. A. et al. The Food and Drug Administration's regulation of tobacco products. *New England Journal of Medicine, 335,* 988, 1996.

McGinniss, M. Personal communication, October 16, 1996.

MacPherson, P. The FDA just says yes. *Hospitals and Health Networks,* May 20, 1996, p. 34.

Mustard, H. S. *Government in public health.* New York: Commonwealth Fund, 1945.

PHF (Public Health Foundation). *Public health agencies 1991: An inventory of programs and block grant expenditures.* Washington, DC: Public Health Foundation, December 1991.

Rawding, N., & Wasserman, M. The local health department. In F. D. Scutchfield & C. W. Keck (Eds.), *Principles of public health practice.* Albany, NY: Delmar, 1996.

Schmeckebier, L. F. *The public health service*. Baltimore, MD: Johns Hopkins University Press, 1923.

Scutchfield, F. D., & Keck, C. W. (Eds.). *Principles of public health practice*. Albany, NY: Delmar, 1996.

Stern, B. J. *Medical services by government: Local, state and federal*. New York: Commonwealth Fund, 1946.

USDHHS (U.S. Department of Health and Human Services). *Healthy people 2000: National health promotion and disease prevention objectives*. Washington, DC: U.S.G.P.O., 1990.

USDHHS (U.S. Department of Health and Human Services). *Fact sheet*. Washington, DC: U.S.G.P.O., March 1996.

USPHS (United States Public Health Service). *Healthy people 2000: Midcourse review and 1995 revisions*. Washington, DC: U.S.G.P.O., 1995.

USPSTF (United States Preventive Services Task Force). *The guide to clinical preventive services*. Baltimore, MD: Williams and Wilkins, 1989.

Weyrich, P. W. The FDA is one of the most irresponsible agencies in the history of our nation. *NetNewsNow!*, July 16, 1996.

Wilson, F. A., & Neuhauser, D. *Health services in the United States*. Cambridge, MA: Ballinger, 1976.

Chapter 7

Principles of Health Planning

BASIC PRINCIPLES OF HEALTH PLANNING

The basic principles of health planning[1] were laid down some time ago and have changed little. Health planning occurs on two levels: macro and micro. The macro level is that of a health services system for the nation, a region, or one or more states. The micro level is that of, for example, an institution such as a hospital or a health maintenance organization; a single, categorical health service provided to a geographic area such as family planning or chronic disease prevention; a health care provider's private office. The primary problem with health planning in the United States is that at neither level are the principles frequently adhered to.

Herman Hilleboe, M.D., one of the primary developers of modern health planning, described the process as follows (1967):[2]

> Planning is an orderly process, put in writing, of:
>
> 1. defining the extent and characteristics of community health problems and identifying unmet needs,
> 2. assessing available and potential resources,
> 3. establishing priority goals (by matching needs and resources and considering alternatives and their consequences),

[1] "Health planning" is a term that subsumes both planning for health maintenance and improvement at the population level and planning for health services.

[2] The reader will notice that many of the references for this chapter are rather elderly. But the thinking they reflect is still right on target, and in any case little new has happened in health planning in the United States for many years.

4. formulating the necessary administrative action to achieve program goals, and
5. relating results to goals by continuing evaluative studies.

Gottlieb (1974) stated three assumptions underlying health planning:

- Resources are scarce; thus ways must be found to secure optimum value from allocations devoted to health.
- Health care serves social purposes and should, therefore, be valued above activity undertaken in pursuit of economic or other social ends.
- An effective health care system is rooted in responsiveness to consumer needs and requires public accountability.

Another developer of modern health-planning approaches, Leonard Rosenfeld, summed up these thoughts well (1968, p. 164): "The aim of planning must be the achievement of optimum use of available resources for the betterment of human welfare."

A contrasting, more contemporary view of the purposes of health planning, eschewing ethical considerations, was offered by Marmor and Bridges (1980, p. 419): "There is a common impetus to health planning in the United States and other industrial countries: the concern to curb rapidly escalating costs." These two views of health planning reflect the current conflict in the managed care realm, to which we have been referring throughout the book and which will consider in more detail in the next chapter, between managed *care* for the benefit of the patient and managed *cost* for the benefit of a for-profit owner.

Types of Health Planning

In their very useful textbook and guide *Basic Health Planning Methods*, Spiegel and Hyman (1978) describe six common types of health services planning, all of which can take place at both the macro and micro levels (p. 11):

- Problem solving planning: Identifying and resolving a specific problem, using the scientific method.
- Program planning: Setting a course of action to deal with a circumscribed problem, usually one that has already been described elsewhere.
- Coordination of efforts and activities planning: Aiming to increase the availability, efficiency, productivity, and effectiveness of various activities and programs.

- Planning for resource allocation: Choosing among various alternatives defined in earlier stages of the planning process in order to achieve the optimal outcome, given limited resources.
- Creation of a plan: Developing a blueprint for action, including recommendations and supporting data.
- Design of standard operating procedures: Creating sets of standards of practice and/or criteria for operation and evaluation.

One or more of these types of planning is part of any health-planning process.

GOALS AND OBJECTIVES

What They Are

Regardless of the type of planning undertaken, to achieve success it is essential that there be stated goals and objectives; that the goals are set forth lucidly; and that the goals are understood and agreed to by all parties concerned. The most frequent cause of failure in planning is neglecting to establish clear, agreed-upon goals and objectives, either as the first step in the process or at least before the program-planning phase (step 4 in the Hilleboe formulation) is begun.

Goals are broad, usually long-range statements of ideal desired outcomes. For example: "All Americans shall have equal access to health care of high quality." Objectives refer to specific targets of action that are considered to be attainable. They are usually to be reached within a named time. The degree to which the planned program achieves its objectives, within the time specified, should be measurable. For example: "Within 10 years there shall be one primary-care practitioner for every 1,000 Americans."

As the planning process proceeds, it may be appropriate or necessary to add to or modify goals and objectives written earlier. This "feedback-loop" mechanism is one of the principal engines of the planning process. Obviously, one cannot write a complete set of goals and objectives before beginning a planning process. In fact, it is often the case that at the beginning one can write only goals, not objectives.

As data are gathered, however—and no planning process can take place without data gathering, whether historical, anecdotal, observational, or numerical—then specific objectives can be defined. The recognition of the importance of data, the adequate gathering of it, and the scientific (as contrasted with, say, the ideological) interpretation of it are all essential to effective, useful planning. Commonly, the more preconceived notions based on ideology are projected into the planning process, the more the process proceeds in the absence of data, an activity known as ''data-free'' planning.

Realism is an essential element of any effective health-planning process and program. First, regardless of the health or health care problem being faced, to make the planning enterprise worthwhile it must be within the realm of possibility that the problem can be solved given present knowledge, personnel, and available interventions. Second, if stated goals are unrealistic (e.g., in dealing with illicit drugs such as marijuana, heroin, and cocaine setting the achievement of a ''Drug-Free America'' as the goal for the ''Drug War'' in a nation of 100 million users of alcohol and more than 50 million users of tobacco is unrealistic) the resultant program will often be incapable of achieving any positive results and may produce negative ones (as is the case of the public policy known as the ''Drug War'' [Jonas, 1995]). Third, realism is also essential for sound priority setting (see Hilleboe, 1967).

Extrinsic and Intrinsic Goals and Objectives

The goals and objectives *of* the planning process are substantive. These can be called *extrinsic*. They define the desired physical and programmatic functional *outcomes* of the endeavor. They describe the reason(s) why the planning process of which they are a product was undertaken in the first place. Examples are: What functions will the new or remodeled building serve? What is the new program for adult screening intended to achieve? What improvements in health care will the reorganization/redesign (mid-1990s buzz word, ''reengineering'') of service ''A'' in the hospital provide for patients?

One can also state goals and objectives *for* the planning process itself. These can be called *intrinsic*. They describe technical planning entities: what kind of product (a report, an analysis, a functional program, a building design, a construction schedule, a personnel recruitment-and-training program) is to be created by when. Intrinsic goals and objectives are used to measure the effectiveness of the planning process on its own terms: were planning meetings held, how many, who participated, was a functional program developed, did the physical plans provide for the spaces required to carry out the functional program, was everything done on time? In planning, the term ''goals and objectives'' usually refers to extrinsic ones. That is the case in the balance of this chapter.

Failure to Define Goals and Objectives

When planners fail to clearly state usable goals and objectives, and this happens with depressing frequency in health planning in the United States, they usually encounter the following pitfalls:

- There is no way to evaluate the effectiveness of the planning process, because what was being planned *for* has not been defined.
- Reams of data are collected, much of them useless because of a lack of focus.
- Inadequate data are collected and decisions are made on the basis of incomplete knowledge and understanding.
- Ideology or preconceived notions is/are used either in place of data or in place of using the scientific method to interpret them.
- Planning for health services *functions* and *operations* is confused with and sometimes superseded by planning for *physical space.*

The development of goals and objectives is sometimes ignored in the planning process, and/or they are sometimes written so vaguely or in such general terms as to be meaningless and useless. Several reasons account for this state of affairs. First, the larger the group of interests affected by the proposed program, the more difficult it is to define goals and objectives that all parties can agree to. It is sometimes easier for leadership to skip this stage than go through the political process necessary to hammer them out.

Second, some of the parties involved may have goals and objectives in mind they feel would not be: (a) accepted under close scrutiny, (b) justified by data collection and analysis, or (c) economically feasible. If such persons are in positions of power from which they can develop and implement programs without setting forth written goals and objectives, they will often do so. Third, the glitter of the *techniques* of planning, the collection and analysis of data, the designing of administrative structures and staffing patterns, the development of budgets, and above all, the laying out of space, can easily outshine the fundamental, unglamorous, at times much more difficult job of determining "Why and for whom are we doing this?"

Function and Form

Often health services planning activity results in a new or remodeled building. It is virtually impossible to design a building to appropriately meet specified health services needs, that is, to carry out a certain set of functions, unless a functional program is established on paper before the building-design process begins. The functional program is a specification of activities, expected clientele, hours of service, staffing requirements and patterns, organizational structure, projected budget, and so on.

To develop a functional program goals and objectives must clearly be defined. However, as noted, this can sometimes be a difficult job. And even when goals and objectives have been properly spelled out, sometimes a functional program is still not developed because that too is a difficult, data-based task. Nevertheless, it often happens that when this essential part of the process is bypassed or done poorly, a building will be designed and built anyway.

In this case, the planners focus alone on the layout of the building rather than on its intended uses. The blueprints show rooms and corridors, doors and windows, closets and conference rooms. But nowhere is there a document that shows, except perhaps in the most general terms, *how* and *for what* these spaces are to be used once they become a reality in concrete and steel. More often than not, then, the building is designed to fit the available land and/or to spend the available money.

Building to occupy available land or spend available money rather than to meet defined unmet needs by achieving specified goals and objectives of course violates Frank Lloyd Wright's elemental architectural dictum: "Form should follow function." In the former scenario, often after construction has started, someone says: "What needs do we meet with this space?" rather than before construction begins posing the question: "What space(s) are required to meet these needs?"

There are numerous expensive concrete-and-steel edifices used only to partial capacity, while community needs for other types of health services go unmet. These structures have been produced by a health-planning process in which function followed form rather than the other, correct, way round.

Planning and Values

In setting goals and objectives, it is important to remember that there is no such thing as "value free planning" (Fein, 1974, p. 67). Every planner and participant in the planning process is influenced by her or his "ideological baggage." The latter affects, indeed determines, one's value judgments and ordering of social priorities. Recall Rosenfeld's (1968, p. 164) statement, quoted in the introduction to this chapter, on the aim of planning: "[It] must be the achievement of *optimum use* of *available resources* for *the betterment of human welfare*" (emphasis added).

The very fact that Dr. Rosenfeld included "optimum use," "available resources," and "the betterment of human welfare" in his description of the aim of the planning process reflects his own values. Further, within Dr. Rosenfeld's description, the concepts of just what constitutes "optimum use," "available resources," and "the betterment of human welfare" will vary from person to person, reflecting differences in *their* values. Even in the presence of scientifically gathered data, each person's social values and priorities will strongly influence the nature of their analysis and use of the information.

Patient Needs and Provider Needs

The workings of the health care delivery system have many different outcomes. Some serve the needs of the people receiving health and sickness care services. Others serve personal, nonhealth care needs of people who work in the system. Meeting these two sometime disparate sets of needs requires establishing two sometimes disparate sets of goals and objectives. Often the goals and objectives of those who work in the health care delivery system are the same as those of the people being served, that is, improving health status and combating disease. On occasion, however, they are not.

Provider needs and goals can be of a different order than those of patients. Consider these goals, for example: power, profits, prestige, institutional preservation and growth, career advancement, intellectual stimulation and development, and political gain. If two sets of goals and objectives exist side by side, spelled out in writing or not, and if there are unresolved conflicts between them, the result often is irrational, or no, planning.

THE HEALTH SERVICES PLANNING PROCESS

Introduction

The basic concepts of health planning set forth at the beginning of this chapter are straightforward. The fragmented health care delivery system in the United States, however, affects the nature of the technical planning process (Tierney & Waters, 1983). The science of planning, as noted above, consists of collecting and using data. The type and quantity of data needed depend on the existing level of health knowledge and planning knowledge, the particular health care delivery component being planned for, and the characteristics of the larger social framework in which it is found.

Without planning data, there is no baseline against which one can measure the impact of implemented programs. To do the latter, information is needed on the extent to which anticipated changes in health status occur, at what cost, and with what positive or negative side effects. Indeed, baseline data provide the foundation for systems of continuous feedback, systems that must be in place if inappropriate goals or inadequate work activities are to be identified and corrected.

When planning is done correctly, that is as a continuous, cyclical whole (Sigmond, 1968), all categories of data are relevant throughout, although one may be used more in one planning stage than in another. Planning for health services requires data on the following:

1. the population to be served;
2. its health status; and
3. existing health care resources and their utilization.

Without such information one cannot determine, for example, whether the expressed *demand* for health services is greater than, equal to, or less than the *need* for health services. "Demand" is a measure of the quantity and quality of health care services that *consumers* want, usually based on subjective evaluations. "Need" is a measure of the quantity and quality of health services that *health professionals* estimate are required, based on various epidemiologic/demographic, health and disease status, and health services use indices.

Measuring Health Status

The first step is to measure health and illness levels in the population to be served. This can be the population of the nation as a whole, of a defined community, or of users of an existing service that is a candidate for redesign. Then the health service needs of the target population can be estimated.

Some illustrative demographic data for the U.S. population is presented in chapter 1. A population's health status is assessed by measures of mortality and morbidity or combinations of the two (Rice, 1994). Traditionally, mortality (overall, maternal, infant, and other death rates) has been the primary indicator of a population's health. Mortality indices, however, are less than optimal measures of health. For example, death is an opposite of health; it is thus only an indirect measure of health status.

Measures of morbidity, the presence of a disease condition or active pathology, and disability, restricted performance of normal functions, perhaps give a better picture of a population's health status, although the parameters are still ones of sickness, not health. In addition, they do present problems of collection and interpretation, as well as others. For example, there are a limited number of legally reportable diseases, and selective reporting leads to inaccurate data (Blum, 1974). Further the definition and classification of morbidity states can be difficult.

Other useful parameters for health planning are the prevalence of various health risk factors in the population, such as cigarette smoking, obesity, and sedentary lifestyle. Planners also measure the health status of a population by its present level of health services usage: frequency, location, who is and isn't using presently available services, intensity of service in terms, say, of diagnostic testing, and so forth. These data are also part of the description of existing resources (see next section).

Describing Existing Resources

The next step is to undertake an inventory and evaluation of existing services (Spiegel & Hyman, 1978). There are three kinds of resources to be described: human, physical, and financial. For personnel, the number, age, sex, education, specialization, type of practice, productivity, geographic location, and availability must be determined, along with the output of operating and approved training programs. Existing sources of care must be inventoried by number, distribution, and characteristics such as size, type, volume, and quality of services offered; condition of the physical spaces used; licensure and accreditation status; policies; financial solvency; and referral patterns.

For each facility, patient characteristics must be described and usage measures compiled, such as number of admissions, average daily census, percentage of occupancy, average length of stay compiled. Financial data concerning, for example, amounts spent, for whom, for what services, from what payment sources (government, private insurance, philanthropy), paid out to whom and how, must be obtained.

Determining Unmet Need

This is the central step of the planning process. The data on health status, even if indirect as they usually are, enable the planners to estimate total health services needs. From the description of and usage data for the available resources, the planners can then estimate the portion of total need that is being met by them. Available resources constitute the supply side of the planning equation: sociodemographic factors, health status measures, and professional assessments of undetected problems describe the demand/need side. The need that is not being met either wholly or in part is called the ''unmet need.'' By using both the available mathematical tools and subjective estimates, the planner weighs one side of the equation against the other, and comes up with (one hopes) a complete estimate of ''unmet need'' (Spiegel & Hyman, 1978).

Program Planning

The next stage of the planning process is creating a program to meet those presently unmet needs. At this point in the process the originally stated goals must be reconsidered in light of the data obtained and analyzed. Goals may remain unchanged or they may be redefined, reduced, or enlarged in scope. Objectives can now be written with more specificity. For a successful outcome, the refining of goals and objectives, after the unmet needs have been carefully delineated and before program planning begins, is critical.

In planning a program to meet unmet needs, the following (similar to the description of existing resources) must be provided for: description of new or expanded services to be offered; personnel requirements and staffing patterns; policy setting and administrative structure and mechanisms; financing systems to raise, budget, and pay out the funds needed for program operation; physical space; and a means for program evaluation and ongoing forward planning. As discussed earlier, in order to have the best chance of creating a service that will truly meet community needs, program planning should always precede physical space planning.

If at all possible before implementation, proposed programs should be tested by one means or another. It is rarely possible in the real world to run a purely scientific, prospective experiment of a planned program before it is fully implemented. It is often possible to undertake a retrospective evaluation of other, similar, previously implemented programs, however. This can be done through the literature, by private mail and telephone surveys, and by direct observation. This kind of analysis, not always done in the real world, can prove to be very useful. Pitfalls can be skirted, ''reinvention of the wheel'' can be avoided, and successful planning and implementation strategies can be adapted to use.

Of course, just because there is past experience with a present policy proposal doesn't necessarily mean that lessons already learned will necessarily be applied to the present case. Take the health care related national welfare reduction act of 1996. Two of the primary arguments for it were that ''high'' welfare payments cause both poverty and illegitimacy.

The fact that the state of Mississippi had both the lowest welfare payments and among the highest poverty and illegitimacy rates (BOC, 1996) seemed to influence the national debate not at all. If widely known and used, the data in this case would have been an inconvenient impediment to ideologically based national policymaking, the latter a clear example of data-free planning. Thus the ideologically and politically inconvenient data were just ignored.

Evaluation

Once implemented, programs should be evaluated. Are the goals and objectives being met? Is the program cost-effective? Are there defects that could and should be remedied? Rossi and Freeman (1993, p. 3) set forth the reasons for doing evaluations: "to judge the worth of ongoing programs and to estimate the usefulness of attempts to improve them; to assess the utility of new programs and initiatives; to increase the effectiveness of program management and administration; and to satisfy the accountability of program sponsors."

Henrik Blum (1974), a long-time health planning analyst, outlined five levels of evaluation:

1. Activity: Is the program operative?
2. Criteria: Is the program operating according to standards (of quality, access, etc.)?
3. Cost: Are program costs in line with those that were agreed on? Can unit cost be improved?
4. Effectiveness: How well is the program achieving the desired output?
5. Outcome validity: To what extent has the program realized the ultimate goal for which it was designed?

It is important to avoid biased measures of outcome. Indeed, the literature on laboratory and field experiments is replete with cautions against evaluator contamination. Program designers are advised against evaluating their own programs, evaluators against implementing their own recommendations. Evaluations can fail in two ways, one of them scientific, the other not. The evaluative methods can be inadequate or faulty, that is, one or more of the five elements of evaluation described by Blum can be missing or incorrectly done. The second "failure" is the inability to produce "acceptable" findings, that is, those consistent with the policymaker's commitment to program success. A planning imperative thus becomes clear. As part of the original planning process a coalition of support for thorough and scientific program evaluation, one that will hold together regardless of political repercussions, must be formed.

A BRIEF HISTORY OF HEALTH PLANNING IN THE U.S.[3]

Early Developments

Historically, recognition of the need for both regional and national comprehensive health planning in the United States can be traced back to the Committee on the Costs of Medical Care, established in 1927, which issued its Final Report in 1932 (see chapter 1) (Committee on the Costs of Medical Care, 1970). An important part of the recommended program was that the delivery of what is now called primary care as well as specialty services be aimed at defined geographic areas and be coordinated within them.

Starting before World War II, there were a few limited local experiments with what was called "regionalization:" the organization of community hospitals and ambulatory care centers around teaching hospitals (Mountin et al., 1945). The American Hospital Association's Committee on Postwar Planning proposed that regionalization be developed on a national basis (Commission on Hospital Care, 1947; see also the Commission on Hospital Care, 1946, on Michigan).

Supported by the Kellogg Foundation, the Commission on Hospital Care issued the following statement in 1947 (p. xi):

> The haphazard development of hospital services of the past should not be extended to the future. The public must be made aware of, must assume its responsibility for the development and support of adequate hospital care on a communitywide basis. The expansion and development of individual institutions must be in accord with an overall planned program for the community. Direct benefits will accrue to both hospitals and public through organized effort in the intelligent planning of hospital care.

The enormous bills for the failure of the nation to heed this advice have come due and will continue to come due for decades to come.

The Hill–Burton Act

The first attempt by the federal government to ensconce health planning into the law came in 1946 with the passage of the Hospital Survey

---

[3]This section is based in part on Jonas, S., Planning for health services, Chapter 15 in S. Jonas (Ed.), *Health care delivery in the United States*. New York: Springer Publishing Co., 1986, pp. 390–403. See also Kropf, R., Planning for health services, in A. Kovner (Ed.), *Health care delivery in the United States* 4th ed., pp. 326–339. New York: Springer Publishing Co., 1990.

and Construction Act, better known as ''Hill–Burton'' after its sponsors, Senator Hill of Alabama and Representative Burton of Michigan. The original stated intent of the act was to improve the hospital bed:population ratio in rural areas and by so doing, among other things, attract physicians to those areas. Federal funds were made available through the states on a matching basis. An important requirement was that each state had to designate a single agency for hospital construction plan development and implementation.

Hill–Burton underwent numerous modifications and expansions of scope. By 1970, the program had assisted in the construction of facilities housing 334,438 hospital beds and 93,749 long-term care beds, as well as 1,032 outpatient facilities, 520 rehabilitation facilities, 1,258 public health centers, and 41 state health laboratories (USDHEW, 1970). In general, the effort was concentrated in areas in which previous shortages had been most acute.

Hill–Burton was limited, however, in that it was a state-based rather than a comprehensive approach to remedying health care inadequacies. It focused overwhelmingly on beds rather than services that might or might not require additional beds. There was little provider–consumer interaction in the program, nor was there much interaction between Hill–Burton activities and other health-planning efforts (Gottlieb, 1974). Finally, because its approach to physician redistribution was all carrot, no stick, its results in that area were less than exemplary (Clark & Koontz, 1973).

Regional Medical Programs

If Hill–Burton was primarily a ''bricks-and-mortar'' program, the Regional Medical Program (RMP) focused on the functional. The law, passed in 1965, was an outgrowth of three of the major recommendations of a Presidential commission headed by Dr. Michael DeBakey (Russell, 1966) (that's the same Dr. DeBakey who advised on the care of Russian President Boris Yeltsin's heart in 1996). President Johnson had charged the commission with developing a ''realistic battle plan leading to the ultimate conquest of three diseases—heart disease, cancer, and stroke'' (President's Commission, 1964).

The original plan called for the development of a nationwide network of ''regional medical complexes'' focused on the three named diseases. Opposition from the American Medical Association, however, caused the insertion into the language of act a prohibition against interfering with ''the patterns or methods of financing of patient care or professional practice.'' That fundamentally changed the focus of what became Public

Law 89-239 from planning and construction to ''volunteerism'' and coordination (Creditor & Nelson, 1975; Jonas, 1967; Komaroff, 1971). The program, expanded in 1970 (Public Law 91-515) to cover all major diseases and negative health conditions, supported continuing professional education, some health services research aimed at coordination of services, and limited direct patient care. It was phased out in the early 1970s.

Comprehensive Health Planning Agencies

In addition to the Regional Medical Programs Act, the 89th Congress passed into law another outgrowth of the DeBakey Commission recommendations, the Public Health Service Act Amendments of 1966 (Public Law 89-749). On paper, at least, it established a system for comprehensive health planning. Included in the law was a statement (see Section 314 [a]) that:

> The Congress declares that fulfillment of our national purpose depends on promoting and assuring the highest level of health attainable for every person, in an environment which contributes positively to healthful individual and family living; . . . Federal financial assistance must be directed to support the marshalling of all health resources . . . to assure comprehensive health services of high quality for every person.

However, a ''non-interference in existing patterns of private practice'' clause was also inserted in this act.

For that reason and others the act failed to achieve its purpose. A complex planning system was established (Hilleboe & Schaefer, 1968; Jacobs & Froh, 1968; Office of Comprehensive Health Planning, 1967; Stebbins & Williams, 1972). The system was so complex on the one hand, and had so little potential power on the other, that little was accomplished during the 8 years or so that it was in existence (Sieverts, 1976). In fact, it could be said that the national government has been in retreat from the lofty goals set forth in the Congressional statement introducing the act since the time of its passage.

The National Health Planning and Resources Development Act of 1974

Late in 1974, the Congress passed the National Health Planning and Resources Development Act, Public Law 93-641. Under it, single state and areawide health-planning agencies were to be created to perform the functions of the Hill–Burton agencies, the Regional Medical Programs, and the Comprehensive Health Planning Organizations created by P.L. 89-749 (Coopers & Lybrand, 1975; Lively, 1978; Rubel, 1976; Werlin et al., 1976; Whiting, 1977). By attempting to end the fragmented approach to health-planning, Congress apparently hoped to realize more than the minimal progress recorded until that time toward achieving stated health and health care delivery goals.

This time, the Secretary of the then-Department of Health, Education, and Welfare was to issue national health-planning goals based on priorities made explicit in the law. State governors were to divide their states into health-planning areas, according to stated criteria. In each there was to be a Health Systems Agency (HSA) responsible for the planning function. HSAs could be public or private nonprofit entities, but not educational institutions, thus excluding the medical schools that had dominated RMP operations.

Under Section 1513 of the Act each HSA was charged with the following:

1. Gathering and analyzing suitable data.
2. Establishing (long-range) health systems plans and (short-range) annual implementation plans.
3. Providing technical and/or financial assistance to those seeking to implement provisions of the plans.
4. Coordinating activities with the Professional Standards Review Organizations (the Medicare quality assurance/utilization review agencies of the time) and other appropriate planning and regulating entities.
5. Reviewing and approving or disapproving applications for federal funds for health programs within the area.
6. Assisting states in the performance of capital expenditures reviews (so-called "certification of need").
7. Assisting states in reviewing institutional health services with respect to the appropriateness of such services.
8. Annually recommending to states projects for the modernization, construction, and conversion of medical facilities in the area.

Except for powers relating to plan development and the disbursement of federal funds, the emphasis was on assisting, recommending, gathering, and coordinating. Nevertheless, the HSA was supposed to carry out the following critical tasks (P.L. 93-641, Sect. 1513 a):

1. Improving the health of the residents of the health service area.

2. Increasing the accessibility, acceptability, continuity, and quality of health services.
3. Restraining cost increases.
4. Preventing unnecessary duplication of health resources.

Duplicating the reality faced by its predecessor acts, however, an incongruity existed in the HSA act between broad goals and limited powers (Jonas, 1975; Shapiro & Russell, 1976; Wildavsky, 1976). Also duplicating previous experience, a complex federal/state/local administrative/bureaucratic system was created for administering the whole thing.

Nevertheless, by the end of 1978 all the state planning bodies, called State Health Planning and Development Agencies, were up and running, as were over 200 Health Systems Agencies. The National Council on Health Planning and Development was functioning, and the first set of National Guidelines for Health Planning had been issued (Foley, 1978; USDHEW, 1978). Their emphasis was on structural elements: bed/population ratios and minimum numerical requirements for various technology-based procedures.

In 1979 for the first time, draft federal guidelines covering the types and characteristics of *health services* goals to be achieved through the health-planning process, were developed (USDHEW, 1979). Also established were specific *health status goals* to be achieved by the health care delivery system. The health services goals were truly comprehensive, covering issues from financial coverage to geographic coverage, from health promotion/disease prevention to the most sophisticated tertiary-care services. Some observers felt that although progress was slow, something was finally happening in comprehensive health planning (Tierney & Waters, 1983).

That progress slowed considerably in the early 1980s, however. The Reagan Administration was totally unsympathetic to this kind of government activity and simply wanted to abolish the whole program (Health Planning, 1981). Even though a Democratic Congress tried to keep it alive, comprehensive health planning aimed at health services eventually died out over most of the country.

Interestingly enough, under the leadership of such visionaries as Dr. J. Michael McGinniss, long-time director of the Office of Disease Prevention and Health Promotion (ODPHP), an active focus on establishing and monitoring progress toward achieving stated health status goals was maintained and indeed flourished. The results of ODPHP's work are still with us in the form of the documents *Healthy People 2000* and *Healthy People 2000: Midcourse Review and 1995 Revisions* that set forth in great detail goals and objectives for the nation's health (USPHS, 1991, 1995).

PROBLEMS AND PLANNING

In 1980 Peter Rogatz, a respected observer of the hospital scene, predicted that the following changes would take place during the 1980s:

- The supply of hospital beds would decrease, the average hospital would increase in size, and hospitals increasingly would offer complex services;
- regulation would become more, not less, a part of hospital life;
- ambulatory surgery would become increasingly common;
- home care services would expand;
- long-term care facilities would increase and special housing for the elderly would become more commonplace;
- hospitals would become increasingly interested in and attached to health maintenance organizations; and
- the hospice movement would expand.

His predictions have proved largely to be correct. The problems and changes have often been dealt with/carried out in a haphazard, uneven, *unplanned* manner, however. A comprehensive health-planning system might well be able to make a real contribution to ensuring that *productive* change takes place. But what is the key to that, and is it indeed possible to find that key in the United States? As noted above, in the past there have been several national health care planning programs in the United States. However, virtually all vestiges of them were swept away by the Reagan Administration to which, it seemed, "planning" was a dirty word. None have returned.

Thus, Dr. Kropf (1990) tells us as the United States entered the 1990s the "federal government provides massive sums of money to be used by state governments, private for-profit and not-for-profit hospitals physicians and other professionals" and "does not, however, have a plan for what services should be provided with the money, how many hospitals should exist and where, or how many physicians should practice in various cities and states."

PLANNING AND PAYMENT FOR SERVICES

Rashi Fein, Chairman of the Institute of Medicine's Committee on Health Planning Goals and Standards, in his preface to the committee's report said that (IOM, 1981, p. iii): "The committee believes that the forces at work in the American health care system, including the various reimbursement mechanisms, cannot be countered by a health planning effort that is divorced, among other limiting factors, from the flow of funds.'' In the U.S. health care system planning has almost never been linked to health services payment, however.

In the mid-1990s, in the context of major change in the U.S. health care delivery system, there is virtually no health services planning going on, whether linked to payment or not. Will that situation change? In 1983, Blum had his doubts:

> Can there be meaningful health planning when so little else is publicly planned? It is my conviction that how health planning is set up is not altogether a result of special interest forces. Its mandate is determined by such societal forces as traditions, socioeconomic political outlooks, formal governance structures, and availability of resources. A society such as ours has strong anticollective biases, fears of government expressed as endless built-in checks and balances, many levels of government, and many regional differences. Thus we will surely require, but have a difficult time developing, a strong national sense of direction that is melded with powerful state if not local participation to allow for ample variation in accordance with local needs and yet falls within nationally set goals. Our planning machinery is likely to be set up in just those ways that have allowed the health sector to create the problems that upset us so. Only under truly stressful shortages of resources, major calamities, or war are major changes going to be demanded of a given sector. That is what we are seeing today, and the official health planning machinery continues very much to one side of the action.

In 1997, at the time of this writing, the situation is no different.

REFERENCES

Blum, H. L. *Planning for health: Development and application of social change theory*. New York: Human Sciences, 1974.

Blum, H. L. *Health planning: Lessons for the future*, by Bonnie Lefkowitz. [Book review.] *Inquiry, 20*, 390, 1983.

BOC (Bureau of the Census). *Statistical abstract of the United States, 1996*. Washington, DC: U.S.G.P.O., 1996.

Clark, L. J., & Koontz, T. L. *Analysis of the impact of the Hill–Burton program on the distribution of the supply of general hospital beds and physicians in the United States, 1950–1970*. Paper delivered at the Annual Meeting of the American Public Health Association, San Francisco, CA, November 1973.

Commission on Hospital Care. *Health resources and needs: The report of the Michigan Hospital Survey*. Battle Creek, MI: Kellogg Foundation, 1946.

Commission on Hospital Care. *Hospital care in the United States*. New York: Commonwealth Fund, 1947.

Committee on the Costs of Medical Care. *Medical care for the American people*. Chicago, IL: University of Chicago Press, 1970. (Original work published 1932.)

Coopers & Lybrand. *Health care in transition*. New York: Author, 1975.

Creditor, M. C., & Nelson, D. Regional medical programs and the Office of Management and Budget—Parallel philosophies. *New England Journal of Medicine, 289,* 239, 1975.

Fein, R. Priorities and decision making in health planning. *Israel Journal of Medical Sciences, 10,* 67, 1974.

Foley, H. A. Assuring the nation's health resources. *Public Health Reports, 93,* 627, 1978.

Gottlieb, S. A brief history of health planning in the United States. In C. C. Havighurst (Ed.), *Regulating health facilities construction*. Washington, DC: American Institute for Public Policy Research, 1974.

Health planning—Saved by the bell? *Washington Report on Medicine and Health/ Perspectives*, July 20, 1981.

Hilleboe, H. E. Health planning on a community basis. Ann Arbor, MI: Delta Omega Lecture, School of Public Health, University of Michigan, July 31, 1967. (mimeographed)

Hilleboe, H. E., & Schaefer, M. Administrative requirements for comprehensive health planning at the state level. *American Journal of Public Health, 58,* 1039, 1968.

IOM (Institute of Medicine, Committee on Health Planning Goals and Standards). *Health planning in the United States: Selected policy issues*. Washington, DC: National Academy Press, 1981.

Jacobs, A. R., & Froh, R. B. Significance of Public Health Law 89-749. *New England Journal of Medicine, 279,* 1314, 1968.

Jonas, S. Heart disease, cancer and stroke—Regional medical programs. *Journal of the National Medical Association, 59,* 7, 1967.

Jonas, S. 74 Planning act is Dubbed "Sleeper:" The perspective from the campus. *The Nation's Health Health, 5*, 2, 1975.

Jonas, S. The drug war: Myth, reality and politics. *Connecticut Law Review, 27,* 623–637, 1995.

Komaroff, A. L. Regional medical programs in search of a mission. *New England Journal of Medicine, 284,* 750, 1971.

Kropf, R. Planning for health services. In A. Kovner (Ed.), *Health care delivery in the United States* (4th ed.). New York: Springer Publishing Co., 1990.

Lively, C. A. P. L. 93-641: A recipe for action. *Hospitals, 52,* 65, 1978.

Marmor, T. R., & Bridges, A. American health planning and the lessons of comparative policy analysis. *Journal of Health Politics, Policy and Law, 5,* 419, 1980.

Mountin, J. W. et al. *Health services areas: Requirements for general hospitals and health centers*. USPHS Pub. No. 292. Washington, DC: 1945.

Office of Comprehensive Health Planning, USPHS. *Information and policies on grants to states for comprehensive health planning*. Washington, DC: Author, 1967.

President's Commission of Heart Disease, Cancer, and Stroke. *A national program to conquer heart disease, cancer, and stroke*. Washington, DC: U.S.G.P.O., 1964.

Rice, D. P. Health status and national health priorities. In P. R. Lee & C. L. Estes (Eds.), *The nation's health* (4th ed.). Boston, MA: Jones and Bartlett, 1994.

Rogatz, P. Directions of the health system for the new decade. *Hospitals*, January 1, 1980, p. 67.

Rosenfeld, L. S. Problems in planning community health services. *Bulletin of the New York Academy of Medicine, 44,* 164, 1968.

Rossi, P. H., & Freeman, H. E. *Evaluation: A systematic approach*. Newbury Park, CA: Sage, 1993.

Rubel, E. J. Implementing the National Health Planning and Resources Development Act of 1974. *Public Health Reports, 91,* 3, 1976.

Russell, J. M. New federal regional medical programs. *New England Journal of Medicine, 275,* 6, 1966.

Shapiro, J. R., & Russell, E. L. P.L. 93-641: Fundamental problems. *New England Journal of Medicine, 295,* 725, 1976.

Sieverts, S. Putting P.L. 93-641 into proper perspective. *Hospitals, J.A.H.A.*, June 16, 1976, p. 125.

Sigmond, R. M. Health planning. *Milbank Memorial Fund Quarterly, 46* (Suppl.), 91, 1968.

Spiegel, A. D., & Hyman, H. H. *Basic health planning methods*. Germantown, MD: Aspen, 1978.

Stebbins, E. L., & Williams, K. N. History and background of health planning in the United States. In W. A. Reinke (Ed.), *Health planning*. Baltimore, MD: Johns Hopkins University Press, 1972.

Tierney, J. T., & Waters, W. J. The evolution of health planning. *New England Journal of Medicine, 308,* 95, 1983.

USDHEW (U.S. Department of Health Education and Welfare). *Facts about the Hill–Burton program, 1 July 1947–30 June, 1970*. Washington, DC: Author, 1970.

USDHEW (U.S. Department of Health Education and Welfare). Health planning: National guidelines. *Federal Register*, March 28, 1978, p. 13040.

USDHEW (U.S. Department of Health Education and Welfare). *National guidelines for health planning (Draft)*. Washington, DC: Health Resources Administration, 1979.

USPHS (United States Public Health Service). *Healthy people 2000: National health promotion and disease prevention objectives*. Washington, DC: U.S.G.P.O., 1991.

USPHS (United States Public Health Service). *Healthy people 2000: Midcourse review and 1995 revisions*. Washington, DC: U.S.G.P.O., 1995.

Werlin, S. H. et al. Implementing formative health planning under P.L. 93-641. *New England Journal of Medicine, 295,* 698, 1976.

Whiting, R. N. The debate continues: Is health planning working? *Hospitals*, April 1, 1977, p. 47.

Wildavsky, A. *Can health be planned?* The 1976 Michael M. Davis Lecture, Chicago, IL: The Center for Health Administration Studies, University of Chicago, 1976.

Chapter **8**

From Group Medical Practice to Managed Care

In October 1996 *Consumer Reports* magazine noted that (''Can HMOs Help,'' 1996, p. 28): ''The public didn't vote for managed care. Nor did its representatives in Congress. Yet HMOs are swiftly reshaping the way Americans get their health care.''

At about the same time, the former Surgeon General of the United States, C. Everett Koop (1996, p. 69), observed:

> The biggest surprise in the past two years has been the rapid growth of a system known as managed care. Millions of Americans have been shifted into health-maintenance organizations, dramatically restructuring the financing and delivery of health care. The original impetus for managed care came from physicians who wanted the freedom to treat their patients without being worried about whether they could pay for each visit, test, or procedure. In the early HMOs, cost containment was an unexpected benefit, not a primary purpose. . . .
>
> But now the rapidly proliferating HMOs—most of them investor-owned and for profit—seem to be interested firstly in managing costs and only secondarily in maintaining health.

Strictly speaking, the term ''health maintenance organization'' (HMO) refers to just one of the organizational forms that is covered by the terms ''managed care'' (MC) and ''managed care organization'' (MCO). As the reader shall see, historically the introduction of the term HMO preceded that of the term MC by some time, and the former described one particular set of health services organizations. The latter has a broader meaning.

In the common health care system parlance of the mid-1990s, however, it happens that the terms are often used interchangeably, as in the *Consumer Reports* quote. Nevertheless, in the text of this chapter "HMO" refers to a specific health care delivery organizational form, described below, whereas "MC" and "MCO" are used to refer to the whole group of organizational forms subsumed under the generic term "managed care," also described below. In other *quotations* in this chapter, however, the reader may well find the terms used interchangeably, as in the preceding quote.

As profit-oriented managed care organizations haphazardly restructure the U.S. health care system in the mid-1990s, Dr. Koop's last observation frames the central question concerning the managed care revolution. As Prof. Dennis Kodner (personal communication, Autumn 1996) has put that question, is it about "managed *cost*" (and potential profits), or is it about "managed *care*" (and potential improvements in quality of medical care)? Aye, there's the rub.

Managed care as a whole, including both the for-profit and the not-for-profit varieties, by the mid-1990s had had a number of positive affects on health and health care in the United States. For example (KPMG, 1996):

- Adjusted for relative risk of death by the relative severity of illness patterns, mortality rates in "high penetration" managed care markets (that is, health services markets with more than 50% of eligible persons enrolled in an MCO) were 5.25% below the national average, even though the former had the highest case severity indices.
- Discretionary hospital costs in high managed care markets were about 19% lower than they were in low ones.
- Patient stays in hospital were 6%–12% shorter than the national average in high and medium managed care markets.
- Hospital costs actually went down in high managed care markets, compared with a 1.44% average increase nationally.

In California, considered the most "mature" managed care market in terms of penetration rate, "between 1983 and 1993 hospital expenditures grew 44% less rapidly in markets with high penetration than in markets with low HMO penetration" (Robinson, 1996, p. 1060).

Managed care also had some negative outcomes. As *Consumer Reports* observed (1996, p. 28):

> [M]any HMOs do offer high-quality treatment. But many people who join an HMO give up a lot: the ability to choose where and how they are treated; longstanding relationships with their doctors, who might not be part of the

HMO; convenient access to care; and sometimes, care that is essential to their health.

Consumer Reports went on to look at the wider health care picture also (1996, p. 28):

> In 1992, *Consumer Reports* argued . . . that the old-fashioned system—based on traditional indemnity insurance and fee-for-service medicine—was in need of change. The system was wasteful and costly, and left too many people without coverage. Then 37 million people had no insurance; today 40 million people have none. But managed care—at least in its current form—does not solve the problems we described.

Nor does it or can it solve most of the other major problems faced by the system: marked geographic maldistribution of facilities and personnel; serious imbalances within the medical profession between specialists and generalists and a probable total oversupply of physicians; an apparent oversupply of registered nurses as the result of purely market-driven changes in the profile of the nursing corps in hospitals; severe lack of attention to both personal prevention and public health; a medical focus on the uncommon but glamorous as contrasted with the common but mundane; an overemphasis on the use of technology and drugs in diagnosis and treatment as contrasted with the use of interpersonal communication and the enhancement of self-efficacy for health; significant deficits in health sciences education and biomedical research policy and practice in relation to public health and health care/services needs, even within the managed care sector itself.

It is in this context, then, that we proceed with our examination of managed care, beginning with its first organizational forerunner, medical group practice.

MEDICAL GROUP PRACTICE

Introduction

Modern MC evolved from group medical practice, a form of physician organization that began in this country about a century ago (Fox, 1996; MacColl, 1966; Mayer & Mayer, 1985). Although solo private practice is still the predominant mode of organization for physicians in the United States, over time group medical practice has slowly and gradually becoming a more common organizational form.

Group medical practice has taken various shapes: private fee-for-service single or multispecialty group practice, prepaid group practice, the health maintenance organization including the Independent Practice Associations (IPAs), and the newer forms of physician association that have appeared as managed care has grown and developed. Other than in the single-specialty variant of private fee-for-service group practice, virtually all groups in the several forms are of the multispecialty variety.

At least five elements of medical practice can be shared in one way or another by a group of physicians: space, supporting staff, practice income, practice expenditures, and the medical work. Many of the numerous possible permutations and combinations of these elements appear in various forms in the U.S. health care delivery system.

Physicians in Group Practice

The American Medical Association defines group medical practice as (AMA, 1996, p. 1):

> The provision of health care services by three or more physicians who are formally organized as a legal entity in which business and clinical facilities, records, and personnel are shared. Income from medical services provided by the group are treated as receipts of the group and distributed according to some prearranged plan.

In 1990, there were about 114,000 physicians working in various types of group practices (AMA, 1990). Some of them worked part time in more than one group, filling about 150,000 medical "slots" in group practices. In 1995 (AMA, 1996), there were close to 20,000 medical groups, up by over 16% from the previous year, with a membership of over 210,000 physicians (some of whom practice in more than one group). Single-specialty groups averaged just over six members (with the subset of family practice groups averaging about 5.6 members), whereas multispecialty groups averaged over 25 members. About 70% of all groups were single specialty, 22% multispecialty, and 8% family practice. In 1995 physicians in group practice comprised more than a third of all nonfederal physicians for the first time. The states with the largest number of groups included California, Pennsylvania, and New York; the smallest number, Hawaii, Alaska, and Vermont.

Private Group Medical Practice

Private medical groups may be single specialty or multispecialty. Single-specialty groups are common in surgery and the surgical subspecialties, obstetrics and gynecology, anesthesia, and radiology, and are found in increasing numbers in internal medicine, pediatrics, and the medical specialties (e.g., cardiology, neurology) as well. In this way the responsibilities for round-the-clock coverage can be shared. There are some private multispecialty groups, but these are less common.

The major advantages of private group medical practice for physicians are: cost sharing of space, support staff, and services; the ability to engage allied health personnel to an extent usually not feasible for the solo practitioner; the sharing of coverage responsibilities for nights and weekends and the ability to readily take vacations and attend academic meetings without having to make special coverage arrangements each time, and ready access to informal consultations when faced with a difficult diagnostic or therapeutic problem.

Prepaid Group Practice

Definition

Prepaid group practice (PPGP) first arose on a very limited basis in the 1890s (MacColl, 1966; Mayer & Mayer, 1985). It took two revolutionary steps. First was the payment to the physicians of a flat fee on a regular basis on behalf of each potential patient to guarantee medical coverage during some specified time period, usually a year, whether or not medical services were used, but regardless of how much medical service was used. The practice of paying a flat fee to a physician to provide a stipulated range of services for the patient for a given time, regardless of how much or how little care the patient needs or uses, came to be known as "capitation" (now one of the two senses in which the term is used [see chapter 5]).

Organizationally linking the payment for medical care in advance of any use with the provision of the medical care itself contrasted PPGP with conventional "indemnity" health insurance (see chapter 5). Under the latter system the insurance company collects money (usually called premiums) from its beneficiaries (actually in most cases the beneficiaries' employers), in advance (as in "prepayment"). The insurance companies then pay for the care that the beneficiaries obtain from whichever sources of care they use, however. Those sources of care are not employed by, contracted to, or owned by the insurer. Under indemnity insurance, payment is made on a *fee-for-service* or *item-of-service* basis, *after* the fact. And there are usually some extra payments ("deductibles" and "coinsurance") that the beneficiaries must make, as well as specified limits in dollars and units/types of service that are covered.

In PPGP the organization acting as the health insurance company also provides the medical care for those persons who are covered. And it usually does this at little or no additional cost to the patient. As the *Harvard Law Review* put it a number of years ago (''The Role of Prepaid Group Practice,'' 1971, p. 901): ''Prepaid group practice may be broadly defined as a medical care delivery system which accepts responsibility for the organization, financing, and delivery of health services for a defined population.'' (The reader will note that this definition is virtually the same as at least the simple ones for an HMO and then MC that we will encounter below.)

Some History

The two major modern major pioneers in this field (there were other smaller ones, too) were the Health Insurance Plan (HIP) in New York City and Kaiser-Permanente on the West Coast (MacColl, 1966). They both were founded during the Depression and then entered periods of significant growth after the end of World War II. As had their early, much smaller, much poorer counterparts in the early 20th century, they encountered much resistance from organized medicine, that is, the American Medical Association and the state and country medical societies.

The resistance was based primarily on an antipathy to the ways these groups paid their physicians. One method was by straight salary. The other was capitation, as described above. Both methods were antithetical to the common fee-for-service, piecework system used by most American physicians. Organized medicine also did not like the idea of contracts between groups of physicians and groups of patients.

Organized medicine always claimed that their opposition to capitation and contracts had nothing to do with money, but with principle. It ''distorted incentives,'' ''made the doctor a wage slave,'' ''interfered with medical judgment,'' ''put a corporation between the physician and the patient,'' ''removed the symbol [the private fee] of the special relationship between doctor and patient.'' As managed care and capitation as the preferred MC mechanism for paying physicians spread, it is unclear whether any of the outcomes that organized medicine predicted would happen as a result are happening, secondary to this increasingly common use of capitation per se. However, it may not be coincidental that physician incomes began to go down (''The Squeeze,'' 1996), at least for the time being.

Forms of PPGP

There are two major forms of PPGP. In the ''staff model'' the physicians work for the organization on a salaried basis. HIP was the classic example of the staff model PPGP. In the "group model" the physicians join together to form their own company. It in turn contracts to provide medical services with the financing and administrative entity that sells the prepaid health care coverage package to beneficiaries and/or their employers. In this case, the physicians' group pays its individual members, either on a salary or capitation basis. Kaiser-Permanente was the classic example of the group model PPGP.

The Advantages of PPGP

As George Silver (1963) and William MacColl (1966) noted back in the 1960s, there are many potential advantages of PPGP. For the physicians they include the opportunity to share knowledge and responsibility, a rational division of labor between generalist and specialist, improved quality of care, regularly allotted time for continuing medical education, a regular work schedule, guaranteed (although not high) income, a fringe-benefit package including malpractice insurance, better access to ancillary personnel and services, and freedom from concern with the business aspects of medical practice.

For the patients, the advantages include no or low charges at time of service, one-stop shopping for 24-hour, 7-day service, continuity of care, and protection against unnecessary hospitalization and surgery. The primary disadvantages for patients center around the possible development of a clinic atmosphere, loss of choice of physician and hospital, delays in receiving service, locational inconvenience, and impersonality.

Historically, the most serious problem with PPGP has seemed to be that they do not often achieve their significant potential for improving the practice of medicine. Dr. E. Richard Weinerman, an early, strong advocate of prepaid group practice, reviewed the experience in 1968 and was disappointed. His observations, although made some time ago, still apply to many current HMOs and other MCOs.

The organizational advantages for the physicians have been implemented, but clinical medicine often remains largely a matter for individual, rather than true group practice. "Group conferences," Weinerman (1968, p. 1423) said, "medical audits and informal office consultations are, in my experience, more common in the descriptive literature than in daily practice." He concluded (p. 1429):

> Perhaps most disappointing has been the hesitation on the part of most medical groups to effect changes in the "way of life" of the medical team itself. This would involve acceptance by the group as a whole of collective responsibility for the health of its patients or members . . . would mean

> actively reaching out into the community for . . . early detection . . . [and] identification and special protection for those at specific risk of disease . . . [and] would imply particular concern for those patients who do not use the service. . . . It implies as much concern with rapport as with diagnostic labels, as much with education as prescription.

Early reflections on the mid-1990s buzz phrases describing the supposed advantages of managed care, "physician–patient partnership," "putting prevention into practice," "make use of community resources," and "work from the epidemiology of the practice," themselves are "more common in the descriptive literature than in daily practice." Thus there is no evidence that, with a few notable exceptions such as the Group Health Cooperative of Puget Sound (WA), much progress has been made along these lines in the intervening years since Weinerman made his somewhat acerbic comments.

HEALTH MAINTENANCE ORGANIZATIONS

Introduction

The trail from PPGP to MC was blazed in part by the health services entity known as the health maintenance organization. (Recall that in the mid-1990s, "HMO" is sometimes used to mean all of the MC forms. As noted, in this chapter "HMO" means HMO as discussed in this section.)

The HMO movement was originally sponsored by the first Nixon Administration (1969–1973). Nixon was interested in the idea because it had been shown that PPGP could save significant amounts of money, primarily by reducing hospitalization (Roemer & Shonick, 1973). Although the organizational *form* produced the desired outcomes, however, there happened to be two problems with using the *name* prepaid group practice to describe what the Administration wanted to do.

First was the name itself. It happened that in attacking the concept and implementation of PPGP over the years, organized medicine had liberally red-baited it and had quite successfully given it a Red label. That was hardly something a President who had first come to national prominence at the height of post-World War II McCarthyite "anticommunism" as a vociferous member of the House of Representatives Un-American Activities Committee would want to be associated with. Second, the developer of the HMO concept, Dr. Paul Ellwood, had in mind not only prepaid *group* practice, but also a prepaid *individual* practice form at first known as the "Foundation for Medical Care," later as the Independent Practice Association (IPA, see below).

Further, although only in the latter stages of development did PPGP take on financial and operational responsibility for hospital as well as ambulatory care, the whole inpatient/outpatient package was built into the HMO concept from the beginning, for reasons of cost-containment if nothing else. Thus, a new name for the old entity with significant new elements had to be found. The name that Dr. Ellwood came up with was "Health Maintenance Organization."

Definitions

A simple definition of an HMO is given by Shouldice (1991, pp. 13, 449):

> An HMO is defined as any organization, either for-profit or nonprofit, that accepts responsibility for providing and delivering a predetermined set of comprehensive health maintenance and treatment services to a voluntarily enrolled population for a prenegotiated and fixed periodic premium payment. [In short], HMOs are organizations that insure groups of individuals against the costs of medical services and also provide those medical services.

This is very similar to the *Harvard Law Review* ("The Role of Prepaid Group Practice," 1971) definition of PPGP, except that group practice per se is not specified.

By the mid-1990s, the Shouldice definition for the most part applied to the totality of managed care and the managed care organization rather than only to the HMO as it was originally conceived by Dr. Ellwood. The mid-1990s reality is rather more complex than the definition described it, however. The modern HMO has a *series* of characteristics that define it. It is the complexity of the present situation that led Prof. D. Kodner (personal communication, Autumn, 1996) to say, "when you've seen one HMO, you've seen one HMO." Nevertheless, while the situation is complex, it is not quite *that* complex and definitions are possible.

One can begin with the "basic five" characteristics of an HMO offered by Harold Luft (1980):

1. The organization assumes contractual responsibility to provide or arrange for a package of health care services, at a minimum hospital care and physician services. The HMO assumes a set of legal obligations, set forth in a written contract that also specifies the premium to be paid for that provision.
2. The organized delivery system serves an enrolled and defined population, with enrollment required for a specified minimum period of time.

3. HMO members are enrolled on a voluntary basis.
4. The HMO receives a fixed, periodic payment, independent of the volume of services provided to each enrollee, from the firm or agency paying for the coverage for that enrollee. This is a "capitated [patient-service] payment" (as contrasted with a "capitated [provider] payment").
5. The provider/financing organization assumes financial risk (that is of a financial loss should the accumulated capitation payments not cover the cost of providing the contracted-for services to all of the enrollees).

In the mid-1980s, Shouldice provided an updated nine-part definition of an HMO (read in mid-1990s terms as MCO) (1991, p. 14): an HMO is *an organized system* that provides *comprehensive benefits* to a *voluntarily enrolled population* living in a *defined geographic area*, that *assumes financial risk*, *accepts prepayment*, uses *medical group practice*, engages in *cost-containment* strategies, and practices *enhanced management* of quality, costs, and patient services through the use of "managing physicians" (otherwise known as "gatekeepers"), and an organizational structure that has "clearly identifiable focal points of responsibility."

When we get to the mid-1990s, however, additional complexities arise that must be taken into account. First, in certain locales there is competition for patients among two or more HMOs. Thus it can no longer be considered that an HMO necessarily serves a defined population in a defined geographic area. Second, the enrollment profile of any one HMO is now constantly changing as employers, and in cases where employees have multiple-choice options, beneficiaries, move from one HMO to another. (Medicare beneficiaries electing to use an HMO may change membership each *month* if they so choose.)

Third, HMO membership is not necessarily voluntary: some employers offer only one health service option to their employees. That is, if the employee wants to take advantage of an offered health care benefit he or she can only use an HMO (rather than a traditional fee-for-service provider) and it must be the HMO the employer selects. Fourth, for any one individual, unless one adopts a very broad definition of "medical group practice," many HMOs cannot be characterized as one.

Complicating the picture even further, certain new organizational forms have been added over the past 15 years. The increasing number of permutations and combinations of the various organizational forms has led to the "when you've seen one, you've seen one" conclusion. Therefore, in addition to the *definition* of the HMO, a *typology* of HMO, and then MC, forms was developed.

The traditional HMO typology, stemming from the early 1970s, reflected the adaptation of PPGP to the HMO model and the addition to it of the Independent Practice Association (IPA). It went as follows (Shouldice, 1991):[1]

1. Staff model. The HMO runs the whole show itself, including employing the physicians and paying them by salary.
2. Group model. The physicians are organized into one or more separate, self-governing multispecialty group practices. They then contract with the HMO to provide the medical services, and the HMO does everything else. The group usually pays its members on a capitation basis, but may use salary or fee-for-service or some combination of all three.
3. The IPA. The physicians remain in their offices, which they *own* and in which they see HMO enrollees. There is no group practice at any level of abstraction and no pooling of either medical or ancillary service resources. The physicians may be paid either on a capitation or fee-for-service basis. The IPA combines solo or small private group practice for the physicians with a prepayment system for the patients. The IPA organizations, as do the group HMOs, operate a central billing and collection system, peer review for quality and utilization of care, and cost-containment mechanisms.

One major difference between group and staff model HMOs on the one hand and IPAs on the other is that the former have ''closed'' medical staffs, that is, the HMO or medical group has full control over its members, whereas in most cases any physician who can meet the (usual minimal) membership qualifications can join an IPA, at his or her option. (It should be noted that although for the most part any physician can *join* any IPA, the medical manager usually has the power to ''deselect'' any physician who does not abide by the IPA's rules and procedures.)

Just as in the mid-1990s there are limitations in the *definition* of an HMO, there are some newer *organizational forms* that this traditional typology doesn't cover either. We will review them below, in the section on managed care.

HMOs Entering the 1990s

Among the developments being undertaken by HMOs as they prepared to meet the challenges of the 1990s were (Belodoff, 1990):

[1]It should be noted that all of these definitions are concerned with *physician organizations only*.

- The introduction of ''point-of-service plans'' allowing members to use nonplan providers by paying an additional fee.
- Increasing cooperation between HMOs and major health insurers like Blue Cross.
- Acceptance of workers' compensation cases.
- Expansion of health promotion/disease prevention, worksite safety, and employees' assistance programs (EAPs serve employees with addictive behavior problems).
- Development of packages focused on the currently uninsured population, should a comprehensive national health program be instituted (see chapter 9).

Also becoming more common in the mid-1990s is the ''Network,'' a hybrid form that usually has at its center an HMO, commonly of the IPA type, and then adds a ''Point-of-Service'' (POS) feature (Hagland, 1996) (see also below). It allows HMO patients to also go outside of plan to providers of their choice. These providers are then paid on an indemnity basis, with the patient bearing a significant deductible/coinsurance burden. That ''Point-of-Service'' plans are on the increase possibly indicates some resistance to change on the part of patients.

MANAGED CARE

Definition

The definition of managed care is one that undergoing constant change. We shall consider several of the principal definitions that have appeared over time. Just as MC itself has evolved from the HMO, so have the definitions of MC evolved from the definitions of the HMO.

Looking at the situation from the perspective of the purchaser of health care (most often the employer who is paying the bulk if not all of the health care premium), rather than from that of either the provider or the patient, Peter D. Fox (1990, p. 1) tells us that:

> ''Managed care'' . . . broadly defined, encompasses any measure that, from the perspective of the purchaser of health care, favorably affects the price of services, the site at which the services are received, or their utilization. As such, it represents a continuum—from plans that, for example, do no more than require prior authorization of inpatient stays, to the staff model HMO that employs its doctors and assumes risk for delivering a comprehensive benefit package. Ideally managed care should not simply seek to *reduce*

costs; rather, it should strive to *maximize value*, which includes a concern with quality and access.

The common techniques that MCOs (and indeed HMOs before them) use to control expenditures are "precertification" for hospital admission and the use of many diagnostic and therapeutic interventions, and what is called case management. Precertification is the obtaining by the responsible physician from some central office of the MCO the permission to proceed along a certain medical line before proceeding. Case management is keeping close track of what is happening to hospitalized patients and making sure that their care and discharge follow along preset lines as indicated by the admitting diagnosis unless there are very good medical reasons to deviate from them.

There are a number of different forms of MCO (Wagner, 1996). The range can be seen as a continuum, beginning with "managed indemnity" (adding some elements of cost control, precertification, and case management to indemnity insurance) and ending up at the other end with the Integrated Delivery System (see below).

- Health maintenance organization (previously covered).
- Preferred provider organization (PPO): a group of independent providers (usually private practitioners or private medical groups) that has contracted with an insurer to provide named services at fixed fees. (Unlike most IPAs, which are also organizations of privately practicing physicians, the PPO does not focus on the provision of primary care/comprehensive care, but is used more commonly for physicians providing diagnostic and therapeutic invasive procedures.) The fees are set below the prevailing market rate. The insurer's beneficiaries are given a list of the "preferred providers." Although the patient does not have to choose a provider from the list, he/she is guaranteed that if he/she does so there will be no or low copayments. The advantage to the insurer is cost savings, to the provider it is a guarantee of work.
- Exclusive provider organization (EPO): similar to the PPO, except that the beneficiary must choose a physician on the insurer's list if he/she is to receive any reimbursement for the costs of care.
- Independent practice association (previously covered).
- Independent practice organization (IPO): similar to an IPA, but whereas in IPAs the physicians deal with one insurer, in an IPO an organized group of independently practicing physicians accepts patients and payments from more than one insurer.
- Physician hospital organization/Combined provider organization (PHO/CPO): a variant of the PPO/EPO/IPA/IPO concept organized

by a hospital and/or its medical staff. There are many possible combinations of insurance mechanisms, administrative forms, benefit packages, use of copayment, and means of physician and institutional reimbursement. They are usually formed to provide a hospital and its medical staff the opportunity to band together to negotiate favorable rates with payors.

- ''Point-of-service'' plans (mentioned above): are variants of all of the above arrangements, which, in addition to the standard package, allow their beneficiaries some use of providers who are outside of the organization. It is similar, in fact, to the PPO concept, except that plans with a POS feature usually attempt to provide a comprehensive package of benefits.

More Questions, More Definitional Complications

In addition to the more complex typology, there are other characteristics that must be taken into account in understanding the field in the mid-1990s. Welch and his colleagues (1990) set forth several questions, the answers to which would improve understanding of the complexity that is MC.

1. Do the physicians in a given MCO see MCO patients only, or do they have a mixed practice?
2. Is there an organizational ''middle tier'' that might process payment, carry out case management and utilization review, handle quality assurance, and possibly offer office management services to physicians in an IPA, standing between the MCO that has the contractual obligation to provide the services (directly or indirectly) to its enrollees, and the individual and institutional providers of those services.
3. Is there a ''withhold'' in the payment arrangement with the physicians (that is, do the physicians not get their full pay until it is clear that certain performance standards, primarily focused on utilization and cost-containment, have been met, usually over the course of a year)?

Hornbrook and Goodman (1991) added two additional important defining questions:

1. Is there *vertical integration* between physicians and institutions and how much (see below, ''Integrated Delivery Systems'')?
2. Is the ownership for profit or not for profit?

Finally, one can consider these additional questions in characterizing MCOs:

1. What is the size of the risk pool?
2. How many providers belong to the MCO?
3. Do individual providers themselves accept financial risks (relates to withholds) and do they routinely buy reinsurance against the possibility that one of their patients might unavoidably require very expensive care for a very serious illness?
4. How does one characterize MCOs serving special needs populations (like the mentally ill, patients with acquired immunodeficiency syndrome [AIDS], drug abusers), Medicare populations, Medicaid populations?
5. Suppose a PPO accepts risk, engages in a contract for total care provision? Is it then an MCO?

Despite the complexity of HMO definition and typology, it appears advisable not to get caught up in minuscule details of definition and typology, unless one is engaged in MC research or is responsible for planning an MCO to be successful in a particular market. There are still four major groups of MCOs: staff-model HMOs; group-model HMOs; IPAs of various sorts; and an expanding category of "other," such as PPOs, PHOs, and networks.

INTEGRATED DELIVERY SYSTEMS

What is called the "Integrated Delivery System" (IDS) is becoming a visible and important element of MC whether it has an insurance function or not. An outcome of the gradual disappearance of traditional fee-for-service private practice, the boundaries that previously existed between physicians and hospitals are gradually disappearing.

A definition of the IDS is offered by Kongstvedt and Plocher (1996, p. 46): "IDSs may be described as falling into three broad categories: systems in which only the physicians are integrated, systems in which the physicians are integrated with facilities (hospitals and ancillary sites), and systems that include the insurance functions."

Formerly, Kodner (personal communication, Autumn 1996) said, "hospitals had doctors; doctors had patients." Now, increasingly, as the various forms of MC spread and take over the health care delivery system, it is the payors, or the insurance, risk-assuming side of the MCO that have the patients, with both the doctors *and* the hospitals providing the health care services for the MCO—and *its* patients.

Shortell and his colleagues (1994, p. 46) define the IDS (and this is in part a *normative* definition, what Shortell et al. would *like* them to be, not necessarily what they all are) as:

> A network of health care organizations that provides and/or arranges a *coordinated continuum* of care to a defined population, and is willing to be held clinically and fiscally responsible for the outcomes and health status of that population [emphasis added].

The elements of the IDS, certainly similar to the HMO, are:

1. It serves a defined population.
2. It provides a defined set of services/benefits.
3. It *integrates services*, administratively and clinically, and has an *integrated information system* covering all of the services offered. These are the elements that distinguish the IDS from the traditional HMO (although certainly an HMO can *be* an IDS).
4. For the most part, payments to providers are made on a capitated basis.

An IDS may have something called a "management services organization" for its physicians. This new entity owns the real estate and other tangible assets of the physicians' offices, and employs their nonmedical staff. The IDS also either owns or operates the hospitals that are part of it. It is projected that a successful IDS in the future will have a minimum of 400–500,000 patients, 275 primary-care physicians, 225 specialists, 900 hospital beds, and one or more long-term care services such as a nursing home or a home health agency. It will pool the funds coming in from several sources. It will have a shared mission, philosophy, and vision. It will have centralized and joint planning and management. It will provide an organized continuum of care, through health care teams.

In short, the *ideal* IDS will provide the type of coordinated, continuous, comprehensive, available, acceptable, and accessible care that was envisioned in the British Dawson Report of 1920 (Sidel & Sidel, 1983), was described in the Final Report of the U.S. Committee on the Costs of Medical Care in 1932, and reappeared in the original bills for what became the Regional Medical Program and Comprehensive Health Planning Acts of 1965 (before, that is, they were gutted in response to pressure from the American Medical Association).

The question in this country still is: Can this sort of care be provided in a system that has *a* primary focus either on physician or corporate incomes/profit accumulation?

MC IN THE MID-1990S

Leading into the last decade of the 20th century, by 1989 there were over 32 million people enrolled in over 600 HMOs of various types (''The Interstudy Edge,'' 1989). More than 40% were in IPAs (which accounted for over 60% of the plans), over 55% in plans with more than 100,000 members, about 53% in plans that were 10 or more years old, about half in for-profit plans (over 67% of the plans were for profit), half in not-for-profit plans.

As of January 1, 1996, HMO enrollment was over 59 million, over 22% of the U.S. population (''How Ranks Grow,'' 1996). There were about 675 HMOs in all (AAHP, 1996). About one third of all commercial MCOs offered managed care to the Medicare population (OMC, 1996b). Most HMO enrollment was in traditional plans, with about 10% in point-of-service plans. The top five HMOs in terms of exclusive enrollment (that is, no POS option) were all in California: the Kaiser Foundation Health Plans of Northern and Southern California, Health Net (CA), PacifiCare of Calif., and FHP Inc. (CA). Additionally, there were over 1,000 PPOs with a membership of over 90 million people (AAHP, 1996).

Of the HMOs, about 15% were owned by a commercial insurance company, 20% by a national managed care chain, 14% by a Blue Cross/Blue Shield company, and 8% each by an individual managed care company or a hospital (AAHP, 1996). Of the PPOs, about 43% were owned by a commercial insurance company, 14% by a national managed care chain, 6% by a Blue Cross/Blue Shield company, and 7% by a hospital, whereas 12% were independently owned (AAHP, 1996).

SOME POLICY ISSUES IN MC

Why Managed Care Now?

There are a variety of explanations for the relatively sudden development of managed care, especially of the profit-making kind. One is that in the mid-1980s, private corporations figured out how they could appropriate for themselves the monetary surpluses generated by the U.S. health care system that traditionally went to the physicians. They did this through a mundane cost-containment intervention called utilization review (UR).

UR had been introduced in the early days of Medicare in an attempt to get control of the major and continuing cost increases generated by the ''usual-and-customary fee'' system for paying physicians that the American Medical Association has extracted from the federal government as its price for going along with Medicare. The open-ended reimbursement system invited both physician overuse and a constant round of gradual increases in those ''usual and customary fees.'' UR, which looked at what physicians were actually doing in terms of utilization of diagnostic and treatment services and hospital lengths of stay for their patients, was one way to do that. (In medicine, utilization of almost any service other than emergency care or a routine office visit is almost always provider, not patient stimulated.)

The way UR originally was used in Medicare, as an after-the-fact review, was not particularly successful. But private corporations saw that if they instituted *before-the-fact* review, the so-called ''management of care,'' and required preuse approval, they could reduce utilization significantly. And that they have been able to do.

In combination with the oversupply of physicians (the product at least in part of the absolute refusal of the U.S. medical establishment to engage in any sort of physician supply planning), and the massive oversupply of hospital beds (the product of the absolute refusal of the U.S. hospital industry to engage in any kind of facilities/services planning), the for-profit MCO industry has been able to institute preauthorization UR on a massive scale, driving down both utilization and prices in the face of facilities and personnel oversupply. At the same time, they have been able to reap handsome profits for themselves and provide handsome incomes for their top executives.

Thus it was this institution of physician-generated utilization controls that made it possible for the for-profits to enter the arena in the direct provision of care. They have been on the relative sidelines up to now, content with pharmaceuticals, hospital supply, nursing homes, and some hospitals. But they have been presented with the opportunity to essentially take that share of the profits that can be generated by the physicians from them and arrogate it to themselves. That is what is now happening.

The Future

A long-time observer of the managed care scene has laid out a list of what he thinks will/should happen over the next 10 years in the managed care industry (D. Kodner, personal communication, Autumn 1996):

1. An increase in the practice of population-based care.
2. An increase in the use of physician/nonphysician team care.
3. The development of highly sophisticated medical, health, and management information systems.
4. The return of physician control.
5. Increased public-sector enrollment: Medicare/Medicaid.
6. "Carve-outs" (health services sectors set outside of the managed care system) for example, mental health, substance abuse, and high-cost subspecialty care.
7. Increased insurance-company ownership of MCOs; insurance companies will get out of indemnity insurance.
8. Decline of both group and staff model plans with a concomitant rise in other forms, such as the IDS.
9. Competition among MCOs on the basis of quality.
10. Going from managed *cost* to managed *care*.

For Profit vs. Not for Profit

Finally, prominent once again is the question of for-profit vs. not-for-profit health care, not just managed care. It is *the* issue at the center of virtually every other issue related to managed care. Profit-making isn't a bad or evil thing per se. The question is not a moral one. It is a functional one. Can a profit-making system and the so-called "free market" solve the myriad major problems of the U.S. health care system, as spelled out earlier in this chapter and elsewhere in this book? Because the focus of a for-profit system must be on profits, by definition, and because the solution of so many of the problems not only cannot generate profits, but also would cost considerable sums of money, the answer would appear to be no.

REFERENCES

AAHP (American Association of Health Plans). *1995–96: Managed health care overview*. Washington, DC: Author, 1996.

AMA (American Medical Association). *Medical groups in the U.S.—A survey of practice characteristics 1990 edition*. Chicago, IL: Author, 1990.

AMA (American Medical Association). *Medical groups in the U.S.—A survey of practice characteristics 1996 edition*. Chicago, IL: Author, 1996.

Belodoff, H. HMOs—New challenges—new products. In National Health Lawyers Association, *The insider's guide to managed care*. Washington, DC: National Health Lawyers Association, 1990.

Can HMOs help solve the health-care crisis? *Consumer Reports*, October 1996, p. 28.

Davis, G. S. Introduction: Managed health care primer. In National Health Lawyers Association, *The insider's guide to managed care*. Washington, DC: National Health Lawyers Association, 1990.

Fox, P. D. Foreword: Overview of managed care trends. In National Health Lawyers Association, *The insider's guide to managed care*. Washington, DC: National Health Lawyers Association, 1990.

Fox, P. D. An overview of managed care. In P. R. Kongstvedt (Ed.), *The managed care health care handbook*. Gaithersburg, MD: Aspen Publishers, 1996.

Hagland, M. Point-of-service: Staying alive. *Hospitals and Health Networks*, October 20, 1996, 58.

HMO ranks grow, profits shrink. *On Managed Care, 1*(2), 1, 1996.

Hornbook, M. C., & Goodman, M. J. Managed care: Penalties, autonomy, risk and integration. In M. Grady (Ed.), *Primary care research: Theory and methods*. Washington, DC: USDHHS/Agency for Health Care Policy Research, 1991.

The interstudy edge. *Medical Benefits, 6*(11), 1, 1989.

Kongstvedt, P. R., & Plocher, D. W. Integrated health care delivery systems. In P. R. Kongstvedt (Ed.), *The managed care health care handbook.* Gaithersburg, MD: Aspen Publishers, 1996.

Koop, C. E. Manage with care. The frontiers of medicine. *Time* [Special Issue], Fall 1996, p. 69.

KPMG (KPMG Peat Marwick LLP). *The impact of managed care on U.S. markets*. Executive Summary, 1996.

Luft, H. Assessing the evidence on HMO performance. *Milbank Memorial Fund Quarterly, Health and Society, 58,* 501, 1980.

MacColl, W. A. *Group practice and the prepayment of medical care*. Washington, DC: Public Affairs Press, 1966.

Mayer, T. R., & Mayer, G. G. HMOs: Origins and development. *New England Journal of Medicine, 312,* 590, 1985.

Robinson, J. C. Decline in hospital utilization and cost inflation under managed care in California. *Journal of the American Medical Association, 276,* 1060, 1996.

Roemer, M. I., & Shonick, W. HMO performance: The recent evidence. *Health and Society, 51,* 271, 1973.

The role of prepaid group practice in relieving the medical care crisis. *Harvard Law Review, 84,* 887, 1971.

Shortell, S. M. et al. The new world of managed care: Creating organized delivery systems. *Health Affairs*, Winter 1994, p. 46.

Shouldice, R. G. *Introduction to managed care*. Arlington, VA: Information Resources Press, 1991.

Sidel, V. W., & Sidel, R. *A healthy state* (rev. ed.). New York: Pantheon, 1983.

Silver, G. A. Group practice—What it is. *Medical Care, 1,* 94, 1963.

The squeeze; managed care's effect on physician earnings. *On Managed Care, 1*(1), 1, 1996a.

Wagner, E. R. Types of managed care organizations. In P. R. Kongstvedt (Ed.), *The managed care health care handbook.* Gaithersburg, MD: Aspen Publishers, 1996.

Weinerman, E. R. Problems and perspectives of group practice. *Bulletin of the New York Academy of Medicine* [2nd Series], *44*, 1423, 1968.

Welch, W. P. et al. Toward new typologies for HMOs. *The Milbank Quarterly, 68,* 221, 1990.

Chapter 9

National Health Insurance and National Health Reform

The term ''national health insurance''[1] (NHI) usually describes a single, countrywide health care financing system run by the government, at one or more jurisdictional levels. With varying prominence over time, proposals to create an NHI system have been on the United States' national political agenda since Teddy Roosevelt made NHI one of the planks of his Bull Moose Party platform in the Presidential election of 1912.

It happened that the Reagan–Bush era (1981–1993) was one in which NHI faded almost completely from the health care political agenda. The prospect experienced a revival during the first 2 years of the Clinton Administration (1993–1994). But with the defeat of what came to be known as the Clinton Health Plan (CHP) (see below), the issue receded again.

Nevertheless, the central problems of the U.S. health care delivery system that any comprehensive NHI program would address, from its

[1]As noted in chapter 1, the term *health insurance* is a misnomer. Generically, insurance is a system that provides for the periodic collection of relatively small sums of money from large numbers of people to protect each of them against the financial consequences of a relatively rare negative event. However, over the course of a lifetime, for most people using health services is *not* a ''relatively rare event.''

Thus ''health insurance'' is not ''insurance'' in the conventional sense. Rather it is a system for the collective, long-term prepayment for the costs of health services. Furthermore, the term is a misnomer also in the sense that not much ''health insurance'' money actually pays for health and its promotion. Rather, most of it goes to cover the costs of care during sickness. Nevertheless, as the term is commonly used, so shall it be used in this chapter.

high cost to the maldistribution of personnel and facilities to the lack of financial access for many people, remain. It also remains true that no fragmented, privately operated health care delivery system can by its nature address most of the major problems in the list. That is so because dealing successfully with most of them would require a comprehensive, coordinated, planned, national approach. Thus, NHI is sure to return as a major political issue. The only question is when and in what form.

THE WORLD HISTORICAL BACKGROUND

The first NHI program appeared on the world stage in the 1880s. (Some might be distressed to learn that both the content and form of the arguments for and against NHI have remained largely fixed since that time. This has been the case regardless of changed circumstances or new information.) It was introduced by Otto von Bismarck, the "Iron Chancellor" of Prussia, and, after 1871, of the unified German state. Shortly after the bourgeois revolution of 1848, he had said: "The social insecurity of the worker is the real cause of their being a peril to the state" (Sigerist, 1960, p. 127). In 1881, the German Kaiser, Wilhelm I, in a speech written by Bismarck, said (Sigerist, 1960, p. 129): "The healing of social evils cannot be sought in the repression of social democratic excesses exclusively but must equally be sought in the positive promotion of the workers' welfare."

From the 1830s onward, various fragmented accident, workers' compensation, and sickness schemes, both compulsory and voluntary, had come into existence in the several German states. Building on them, in 1883 Bismarck succeeded in ushering through the German Reichstag (Parliament) a Sickness Insurance Act (Sigerist, 1960, pp. 121–131). Bismarck had wanted a uniform, national system, excluding those of the existing "sickness societies" that were for profit, retaining only the not-for-profit ones. Understandably the former objected to the prospect of being put out of business. (In this regard they had much in common with the present U.S. health insurance companies. Understandably as well, they protest strongly against any proposed U.S. NHI plan that has no, or a limited, role for them.)

Bismarck settled for a plan that used the then existing network of sickness societies, both for and not for profit. Nevertheless, it was a national program that paid for medical care and provided cash support during periods of sickness and accidental injury for certain categories of workers. Two thirds of the premiums were paid by the employees, one third by the employers. Thus it came to pass that the world's first national health insurance scheme was created, not by a progressive democratic or socialist government, but by a conservative monarchy.

By the 1920s most of the European industrialized countries and Japan had some kind of national health insurance system. In each it usually began as a partial and/or voluntary system, generally then progressing to a comprehensive and compulsory one (Douglas-Wilson & McLachlan, 1973; Fry & Farndale, 1972; Glaser, 1978; Roemer, 1985). After World War II, the English-speaking British Commonwealth countries gradually followed suit (Fry & Farndale, 1972; Lynch & Rapheal, 1963; Roemer, 1985). The United States is the only industrialized country in the world, other than South Africa, not to have some sort of NHI system (Roemer, 1991).

THE HISTORY OF NHI IN THE UNITED STATES

The Early Days

The first campaign for a national health insurance program in the United States was undertaken by the American Association for Labor Legislation (AALL), a middle-class, liberal, reform-minded group founded in 1906 (Anderson, 1968; Burrow, 1963, 1977). As noted, proposals for a broad social insurance plan were part of Teddy Roosevelt's Bull Moose (third) Party platform in 1912 (Burrow, 1963). In 1916 the AALL put forward a standard bill for compulsory medical care and sickness benefits insurance. The AALL proposed that the several states each adopt the program independently. It would have covered persons earning below a certain income level and would have used existing insurance carriers. Employers, employees, and the states would have shared the costs (Anderson, 1968; Burrow, 1963).

At first, support was widespread, extending to the American Medical Association and even the National Association of Manufacturers (Burrow, 1963). Beginning in 1917, however, when the U.S. entry into World War I generally deflated the Reform Movement of the time, opposition began to surface from several quarters. Among the opponents were the American Federation of Labor and the commercial insurance industry (Anderson, 1968; Burrow, 1977).

A battle ensued over the issue within the AMA (Anderson, 1968; Burrow, 1963). As part of an overall shift of power from the academic wing of the medical profession to the practitioner wing, the latter, conservative, faction won out (Harris, 1966).[2] In 1920, the AMA House of Delegates passed the following resolution (Burrow, 1963, p. 150):

> Resolved, that the American Medical Association declares its opposition to the institution of any plan embodying the system of compulsory contributory insurance against illness, or any other plan of compulsory insurance which provides for medical service to be rendered contributors or their dependents, provided, controlled, or regulated by any state or the Federal government.

In toto, that remained the AMA's position until the late 1960s (Harris, 1966). Even in the mid-1970s, by which time the AMA had adopted an NHI proposal of its own that ran counter to the bulk of the 1920 resolution, the "noncompulsory" principle was retained (Committee on Ways and Means, 1974). It was not until 1990 that the AMA had dropped the noncompulsory principle as well (AMA, 1990).

During the New Deal and Its Aftermath

Serious consideration was next given to national health insurance during the development of the Social Security Act of 1935. This consideration was stimulated in part by the Final Report of the Committee on the Costs of Medical Care (1932, 1970; see also Anderson, 1968; Stevens, 1971). In 1934, President Franklin Roosevelt created the Committee on Economic Security to consider the whole question of social insurance. NHI was on the agenda. It did not last long there.

The principal opposition again came from the AMA (Burrow, 1963). Economic Security Committee Executive Director E. E. Witte wrote (Anderson, 1968, p. 108):

> When in 1934 the Committee on Economic Security announced that it was studying health insurance, it was at once subjected to misrepresentation and vilification. In the original social security bill there was one line to the effect that the Social Security Board should study the problem and make a report thereon to Congress. That little line was responsible for so many telegrams to the members of Congress that the entire social security program seemed endangered until the Ways and Means Committee unanimously struck it out of the bill.

[2]Both Burrow's book and the Harris, 1966 articles contain detailed histories and analyses of the AMA's involvement in legislative battles over NHI. The Burrow's (1963) book detailed these battles through the 1950s. The Harris (1966) articles covered the Medicare struggles. An excellent overall historical perspective was provided by Falk (1977).

The President wanted to make sure that the basic Social Security Act, conceived as one of the cornerstones of the New Deal, became law. It was eventually passed by Congress with no reference to NHI.

Senator Robert F. Wagner, Sr. of New York State initiated the next major legislative foray on behalf of NHI in the United States.[3] His landmark Wagner (National Labor Relations) Act of 1935 had established the right to collective bargaining for all nonpublic employees in the United States. In 1939, he introduced a bill (Sigerist, 1960, pp. 189–190):

> to provide for the general welfare by enabling the several states to make more adequate provision for public health, prevention and control of disease, maternal and child health services, construction, and maintenance of needed hospitals and health centers, care of the sick, disability insurance, and training of personnel.

The bill, S. 1620, proposed to subsidize: state public health programs (this later became federal policy through a series of separate acts), the construction of hospitals (enacted in 1946 as the Hill–Burton Act), and state programs for medical care for the poor (eventually enacted in part in 1960 as the ''Kerr/Mills'' Medical Assistance for the Aged, then expanded as the federal/state program Medicaid, in 1965). The bill also proposed to provide cash sickness benefits (a standard feature of the European/Japanese approach to NHI that has never made headway in the United States). As well, there was to be a program of federal subsidies to those states enacting comprehensive health insurance programs (Harris, 1966; Sigerist, 1960). The bill died in committee, after being vigorously attacked by the AMA (Harris, 1966).

Senator Wagner tried again in 1943, this time in concert with Senator Murray and Representative Dingell (the father of the current Representative Dingell of Michigan). Their S. 1161 ''advocated a national (i.e., federal) compulsory system of health insurance, financed from payroll taxes and providing comprehensive health and medical benefits through entitlement to ''specified medical service benefits'' (Stevens, 1971, p. 272). This was the first major legislative proposal for a federal rather than a state-based system.

Once again, the AMA responded, negatively, with vigor (Harris, 1966). The bill never got very far, although it was reintroduced in several successive Congresses (Anderson, 1968). In 1947, Senator Robert Taft, Sr.

---

[3]The details of all major NHI proposals made between 1935 and 1957 were summarized by A. W. Brewster, *Health insurance and related proposals for financing personal health services*. Washington, DC: U.S.G.P.O., 1958.

introduced the first Medicaid-like proposal for federal subsidies to the states to pay for medical care for the poor (Stevens, 1971). Though sponsored by a conservative Republican, it also got nowhere.

In 1949 Harry Truman was reelected President with Democratic majorities in both houses of Congress. He decided to make enactment of NHI a major goal of his Administration. He proposed a national, compulsory system, to be paid for by a combination of Social Security and general taxation, similar in many ways to the Wagner–Murray–Dingell bill of 1943. It was in 1945 that Truman had first enunciated the principles on which the proposed system would be based (Committee on Medical Care Teaching, 1958c, pp. 629–630):

> Everyone should have ready access to all necessary medical, hospital, and related services. . . . A system of *required prepayment* would not only spread the costs of medical care, it would also *prevent* much serious disease. . . . Such a system of prepayment should cover medical, hospital, nursing, and laboratory services. It should cover dental care [as far as] resources of the system permit . . . the nation-wide system must be highly decentralized in administration. . . . Subject to national standards, methods and rates of paying doctors and hospitals should be adjusted locally. . . . *People should remain free to choose* their own physicians and hospitals. . . . Likewise *physicians should remain free to accept or reject patients*. . . . Our voluntary hospitals and our city, county, and state general hospitals, in the same way, must be free to participate in the system to whatever extent they wish. . . . What I am recommending is not socialized medicine. Socialized medicine means that all doctors work as employees of government. . . . No such system is proposed [emphasis added].

Does this statement not have a highly contemporary ring to it?

The AMA mounted a furious attack on the plan, based primarily on the thesis that it was indeed "socialized medicine" (Harris, 1966). The AMA used a major public relations firm and a war chest of over $2 million, a very substantial sum in those days. With allies from the drug and insurance industries (Stevens, 1971), it was once again successful in defeating an NHI plan in Congress. With the election of a Republican government in 1952, the AMA was able to breathe easily (Burrow, 1963).

In the post-World War II climate of domestic and foreign anticommunism (Freeland, 1975), it was difficult for Truman to win support at home for a program consistently attacked as "communist" or "socialist," but in any case "red" (Harris, 1966). Thus, in 1951, on the recommendation of Oscar Ewing, the then federal Security Administrator, the Truman Administration withdrew its support for NHI and began the campaign that eventually led to the passage in 1965 of Medicare, limited health insurance for the aged (Harris, 1966; Stevens, 1971).

Medicare and Medicaid

The campaign for Medicare was long and arduous (Harris, 1966; Stevens, 1971). It and its afterthought companion, Medicaid, (Friedman, 1977) finally were passed by Congress in 1965 (Committee on Finance, 1970). Both had their historical antecedents, as previously noted. For example, the earliest AALL proposals contained the concept of beginning with partial coverage, aimed at the working poor. (In contrast, Medicaid covers primarily the nonworking poor.) Medicaid-like proposals had appeared in Senator Wagner's prewar bill and Senator Taft's postwar bills. Determination of an eligible population by age as in Medicare was, however, a relatively new twist, going back only to 1950. However, failing to follow the example of the world's other industrialized countries, since 1965 the progression from some sort of partial coverage to comprehensive coverage, or close to it, just has never taken place in the U.S. That has not been because of a lack of trying on behalf of the reform forces, but rather because of the strength of the political and health care system opponents of such change.

National Health Insurance in the 1960s and 1970s

Once Congress had passed Medicare and Medicaid, beginning in the late 1960s many new legislative proposals for NHI were made, (Burns, 1971; Eilers, 1971; Falk, 1973, 1977; New York Academy of Medicine, 1972). In the 1970s they were summarized by the Ways and Means Committee of the House of Representatives (e.g., Committee on Ways and Means, 1974), the Senate Finance Committee (Committee on Finance, 1979), and Karen Davis (1975). As noted above, in the wide-ranging debate on NHI the basic arguments of the several sides had changed little over time (Committee on Medical Care, 1958a, 1958c; Falk, 1973; H. Schwartz, 1972).

As of 1975, a time when the passage of some sort of NHI seemed imminent to many observers, there were four major proposals before Congress. The constituencies represented were: organized labor, the American Hospital Association, the Health Insurance Association of America, and, notably, the AMA itself. Because all of the major actors were on stage, it was believed that surely one of these proposals or some compromise among them would find its way through Congress.

One predicts the passage of National Health Insurance in the U.S. at one's peril, however. For example, in 1974, an observer wrote (Jonas, 1974, p. 143):

> The United States of America is the only major country in the developed, capitalist world without some form of national health insurance programme. The struggle for national health insurance in the U.S., a long and bitter one, has been well described. It now appears as if there will be some form of national health insurance legislation in the U.S. *before the Presidential elections of 1976* (emphasis added).

There wasn't.

In the 1976 Presidential campaign, Candidate Jimmy Carter said, in his only speech on health policy (''Insurance Plan Stresses Reform,'' 1976, p. 7):

> We must have a comprehensive program of national health insurance. . . . The coverage must be universal and mandatory. We must lower the present barriers, in insurance coverage and otherwise, to preventive and primary care and thus reduce the need for hospitalization. We must have strong cost and quality controls, and . . . rates . . . should be set in advance. . . . We must phase in the program as rapidly as revenues permit, helping first those who need help, and achieving a comprehensive program well defined in the end.

Carter's Administration never submitted such a proposal to Congress.

National Health Insurance Proposals in the 1980s

In 1979 the Congressional Research Service of the Library of Congress (Cavalier, 1979) stated that the major policy issues to be addressed in designing and NHI program were as follows:

1. The rising costs of health care.
2. The gaps in present health insurance coverage, in terms of both services and populations.
3. Geographic maldistribution of personnel and facilities.
4. Access to health care service by ability to pay, social class, age group, and geography.
5. The impact or lack thereof of NHI on the population's health status.

Once again, this list, published close to 20 years before the publication of this book, has a familiar sound to it. It still describes the major problems facing the nation's health care delivery system. In 1980, the same major NHI-proposal players were still on the field (Committee on Finance, 1979; Jonas, 1981a; Kimble, 1979). But with the election of Ronald Reagan in 1980, the whole movement just ran out of gas.

A measure of the enormous loss of energy suffered by the pro-NHI forces in the 1980s can be found in the contents of the "reform package" offered in 1985 by Senator Kennedy (with Representative Fortney "Pete" Stark, House Ways and Means Committee Health Subcommittee Chair). They proposed ("Stark, Kennedy to Propose," 1985):

1. To reduce the number of persons uninsured for health care costs by requiring employers to make health insurance available to former employees at group rates.
2. To reduce or eliminate "patient dumping" by hospitals.
3. To restrain increases in Medicare Part A premium costs.
4. To hold down Medicare payments to hospitals.

This was a far cry from the sweeping changes proposed by Kennedy in several of the major bills he offered in the 1970s. (That weak cry of 1985 had an echo in 1996 with the eventual passage of a bill sponsored by Senators Kennedy and Nancy Landon Kassebaum that provided that certain elements of portability become required for employer-provided health insurance.)

SOME CONTEMPORARY APPROACHES TO NHI

NHI by Contract, or the "Personal Health Care System"

In the early 1980s a proposal designed to deal with the problem list set out by the Congressional Research Service and many others was published (Jonas, 1981b, 1984). First designated "NHI by contract," it was later called the "Personal Health Care System" (PHCS). By 1997 it had yet to be put into legislative language per se, although some of its central concepts appeared as essential elements of the Clinton Health Plan (see below).

The contract mechanism is the classic approach to the achievement of stated goals and objectives. The buyer and seller of a product agree on product or service specifications and costs, written down in a contract. The contract usually contains means of enforcement of its terms. A small-scale, partial prototype of such an approach to the financing, planning, and evaluation of health services (known colloquially as "ghetto medicine") existed in New York City during the 1970s (Jonas, 1977).

Under "NHI by contract," the PHCS would raise the funds necessary to pay for health services, from a variety of sources: general and special taxation, employer/employee contributions, direct payments. It would also be responsible for negotiating a series of contracts with providers. The latter would agree to offer a set of services to the population for a given dollar amount. Most existing providers, whether institutional or individual, would be eligible to become either primary contractors or subcontractors. In this, the PHCS has much in common with the Health Care Corporation concept of the mid-1970s, an American Hospital Association plan, dubbed "Ameriplan" (McMahon, 1975).

The composition of the service packages would be determined by health planning mechanisms. There would be free competition among the providers for the contracts, with bidders offering to provide the specified services at varying prices. Primary contractors would be paid on a global budget basis. Much as MCOs do now, all contractors would then market their services to consumers.

All persons would be covered by a benefit package that would be determined nationally. Consumers would have free choice for contracting with a provider. But once having made a choice, as in present multiple-choice situations, patients would have to stay with the selected provider for some minimum period of time.

Advisory boards consisting of patients served by each contractor would be formed. The consumer role would focus on the evaluation of outcomes, that is, the extent to which contractors met their contract specifications. The boards would be party to contract negotiation and enforcement. There would be graded financial penalties for failure to meet contract specifications, and rewards for excellent performance. Private ownership of the health services sector, including private medical practice, would be maintained. But the people, through both the government and the advisory boards, would have a strong voice in deciding how their money would be spent.

Government responsibilities would be distributed among the national, state, and local jurisdictions. Technology assessment, carried out at the federal level, would provide important data for health planning and priority setting. Insurance companies could be used as fiscal intermediaries.

The PHCS would provide the opportunity to deal directly with most of the principal problems presently facing the U.S. health care delivery system: including cost containment; quality improvement; implementing a comprehensive health promotion and disease prevention program; introducing rationality into the planning, development, and use of personnel and physical resources; and achieving equity of access. The PHCS would leave behind the present reliance on regulation and prayer to achieve program goals and objectives. It would enable the direct focusing of effort and payment, with a fair degree of fine tuning.

The rationale for the PHCS does not begin with benefit packages and decisions on copayment, as do so many other approaches to NHI. Rather it starts with the establishment of planning principles. It assumes that benefit packages will be developed and decisions on copayment made after needs are assessed, goals and objectives are set, and the amount of available funds is determined. Then the contract specifications will be written, balancing needs, priorities, and available funds.

The PHCS would provide an integral link between the planning and financing of health services. As Rashi Fein, Chair of the Institute of Medicine's Committee on Health Planning Goals and Standards noted, in his Preface to the Committee's *Report*, this is essential to problem solving (IOM, 1981, p. iii): "The committee believes that the forces at work in the American health care system, including the various reimbursement mechanisms, cannot be countered by a health planning effort that is divorced, among other limiting factors, from the flow of funds."

Using epidemiological methods in health services planning, the PHCS would carry out ongoing needs assessments, set priorities based on them, and, within the limits of available resources, make continual program adjustments to meet identified needs. The approach would allow for the direct application of planning information to health services system operation. Thus the focus on meeting identified needs could always be maintained without direct government services operation.

An assumption underlying the PHCS approach is that the numerous individual health care providers are, by the very nature of their separateness and independence from one another, incapable of collectively engaging in rational, *comprehensive* planning on their own. The U.S. history of "voluntarism" in health planning and what is happening in the completely unplanned, privately driven, pell-mell rush to managed care have shown that this is true. Thus, if comprehensive health planning is to be carried out, and if health care planning is to be linked with health care financing, government will have to take the lead.

The PHCS concept was developed before managed care became a major player in the system. Because it is at its core a sophisticated health care planning system, however, the PHCS could work equally well with the fee-for-service/indemnity insurance that predominated when it was originally conceived, or with managed care.

National Health Insurance in the Early 1990s

For a variety of reasons (primarily continually escalating costs, a growing pool of uninsured persons, and declining health for certain portions of the population [see also the health care delivery system problem list in chapter 1]), in the early 1990s NHI reappeared with prominence on the national political agenda.

Once again, there were a whole series of proposals placed on the table, from such disparate groups as Senator Kennedy's Committee on Labor and Human Resources (1988); the National Association of Manufacturers (1989); the Heritage Foundation (1989); the National Leadership Commission on Health Care (cochaired by former Presidents Nixon, Ford, and Carter, 1989); the Oil, Chemical, and Atomic Workers (1989); the Committee for National Health Insurance (affiliated with the AFL-CIO; 1989); the American Medical Association (1990); the American Public Health Association (''Insurance Plan Stresses Reform,'' 1990); the U.S. Bipartisan Commission on Comprehensive Health Care of the U.S. Congress (also known as The Pepper Commission; 1990); and the Physicians for a National Health Program (Grumbach et al., 1991; Himmelstein & Woolhandler, 1989).

A number of observers of the U.S. health scene such as Drs. Grumbach, Himmelstein, and Woolhandler have considered the Canadian experience to be instructive.

NHI in Canada

Certain authorities believe that the Canadian experience has much to teach Americans (GAO, 1991, 1992; Woolhandler & Himmelstein, 1989a). What eventually became a national health insurance program for Canada began in one province, Saskatchewan, in 1947 (Lyons, 1996). Nationwide coverage for hospital care was introduced in 1957, followed by coverage for physicians' services in 1971. The Canadian experience with NHI has generated much interest in the U.S., both pro and con (Evans et al., 1989; Fuchs & Hahn, 1990; Goodman, 1989; Igelhart, 1986, 1990; Linton, 1990; ''The Delivery Challenges,'' 1990; Woolhandler & Himmelstein, 1989b).

The present Canadian system has been in place for over 20 years (Roemer, 1991). It was founded on the following four principles:

1. There shall be universal coverage for all Canadians, with low or no copayments, and reasonable access to care.
2. The benefits for each covered person shall be portable from province to province.
3. All medically necessary services shall be covered.
4. Administration shall be by not-for-profit, public agencies.

In practice, this means that all acute care and certain long-term care services are covered. The program is funded primarily from progressive taxation at both the federal and provincial levels. Several provinces do charge premiums, either at a flat rate or in proportion to wages (up to a maximum).

Most hospitals are private and not for profit. The plans pay the hospitals with a lump-sum budget to cover all operating expenses. Capital funds come from the insurance fund, but are allocated to hospitals separately from their expense budgets. (In that way, the plan keeps control of hospital capital expenditure, an essential element of any effective cost-containment program.)

Physicians are paid on a fee-for-service basis, according to a fee schedule negotiated between the provinces and the medical societies. They can bill only for their personal services, not the capital costs of machinery in their private offices or the work of other health professionals. Physicians also cannot "balance-bill" (that is, charge a patient extra for any service covered by the plan). In American terminology, Canadian physicians must "accept assignment" (that is, agree to be paid entirely by the plan, not the patient).

Patients have freedom of choice of provider. Access to care has improved dramatically over the years. Most measures of health are as good or better than those in the United States. Cost increases have been relatively modest (Evans et al., 1989). In the 1960s, the percentage of the gross national product (GNP) spent for health care was about the same in Canada and the U.S. By 1994, it was about 45% higher in the United States.

Of course there are problems with the Canadian system. There has been some rationing (some call it "prudent use") of certain high-tech services. There has been some overservicing by physicians (responded to by the institution of a total income pool and physician income caps). There is some geographic maldistribution of physicians, but it has reduced. (Responses to that problem have been the two tried and true methods of national health care systems: bonuses for going to underserved areas and banning from overserved areas.) Long-term care is uneven among the provinces, but generally it has improved. Prevention still does not receive adequate attention, although its status is better too. The nurse/population ratio is the highest in the world. Thus there is little use of allied health professionals. More threatening in the long-run, however, is the fact that in the 1990s, conservative governments in several of the provinces have been cutting back on funds provided to the health service, even as the proportion of the gross domestic product (GDP) spent on health care has fallen slightly ("Canada's Threatened," 1995; Nolan, 1997).

The major lessons to be learned from the Canadian experience with NHI (at least until it came under assault from the political Right) are not the details of the system (what level of government runs it, who administers it, exactly what the benefits are, exactly what the sources of revenue are, exactly how services are billed for, and so forth).

They are, first, that government has a major role to play in the operation of any smoothly functioning health care delivery system, although government certainly does not have to own and run it to make good things happen. Both ownership and operating responsibility can remain in private hands, as long as everyone is on the same page and government sets the priorities and assembles and allocates the resources at the macro level (rather than having the "free market" attempt to carry out those functions, a role for which it is ill suited as experience has shown us).

Second, we should learn that if changes we make are to have any utility, we must first determine and analyze the true causes of the problems we are setting out to solve. We must aim our solutions at those causes, as the Canadians have done. U.S. reformers only weaken their position by extolling the virtues of the Canadian system to the extent that they must spend most of their time defending that system. Rather, it appears to be more useful to undertake a causal analysis of the problems in the U.S. system, and develop *U.S.* solutions to them. The Canadian experience can then be used as a guide to *how* to solve the problems, not necessarily *what* the specific solutions are. The problem-oriented rather than the detail-focused approach might have benefited the Clinton forces when they put their plan before the public and the Congress in 1993.

The Clinton Health Plan

The Context: Change Was Already Coming

In 1994 the year that the Clinton Health Plan was debated and defeated in the U.S. Congress (Skocpol, 1995), some form of managed care was already the reality for an increasing number of Americans, providers and patients alike (Freudenheim, 1994). Many of the changes that concerned providers the most, including being forced into some form of organized practice and seeing significant declines in their incomes were happening whether or not the CHP or any of the other proposals then on the table were to be enacted. Many managed care induced changes affecting patients, like limiting their choices of plans and providers, were also already a reality for many. Many changes affecting *both* patients and providers, like having insurance/managed care company representatives at the other end of an 800 line making treatment choices, were already a reality too.

One real choice facing the country as a whole at the time of the debate of the CHP was whether this process should occur in a haphazard, unplanned way, or be accomplished in a rational manner. In the latter case, the aim would be to achieve stated goals related to the health and health care of the people, not arising from the narrow interests of the insurance and managed care companies, many of them for-profit, and the provider networks. Another real choice was whether a system heavily dependent on public funds for its operations, like the health care delivery system, should have a strong, on-line public voice in determining its policies and practices. The highly political nature of the debate on the CHP that ensued (Hacker, 1996) ensured that fundamental public policy questions like these would never get a hearing.

The Clinton Health Plan: An Overview

The Clintons' proposed Health Security Act had five primary features: guaranteed private insurance for everyone, choice of physician and health plan, elimination of unfair insurance practices, preservation of Medicare, health benefits guaranteed through the worksite (*Health Security*, 1993). The Act would be based on six basic principles: security, savings, simplicity, choice, quality, and responsibility (*Health Security*, 1993).

One of the CHP's principal public spokespersons, Dr. Irwin Redlener (1993), offered "11 Points" in describing/defending the Plan.

1. It provided for a major overhaul based on the assumption of universal coverage.
2. The plan created a federal framework with state adaptability.
3. It offered a standardized national benefits package, to be prepared, reviewed, and modified from time to time by a National Health Board.
4. It would be paid for by employer/employee contributions, special taxes (much as is done today), and internal savings in the system, primarily by a sharp reduction in the administrative costs of the current highly fragmented and markedly redundant revenue raising/payment mechanisms.
5. The Plan would eliminate employer choice of an employee's health for that employee.
6. The Plan would provide for health care coverage to be transportable from job to job, from health to sickness, from illness to illness.
7. The Plan would create a new system of regional health plans (networks) for the provision of health services and not just a proliferation of HMOs.
8. It would enable patients to make informed choices from among the plans, with the help of objective information provided by the Health Care Alliances (see below).

9. It would improve medical care quality and reduce paperwork.
10. It would make significant changes in the public health system.
11. It would make significant changes in academic medicine.

How the Clinton Health Plan Would Have Worked

A new series of agencies, called Health Care Alliances, would be established by the states. Among other things, as noted by Dr. Redlener, they would collect all of the money used to support health services from all sources. They would then contract with provider networks and groups in their region to provide a package of health care services for all persons enrolled (much like the approach of the PHCS).

The Alliances would have oversight for all quality assurance activities. It would presumably simplify both money flow and paperwork. It would guarantee a choice of plan and a system of quality assurance for the beneficiaries. For the providers it would reunify authority and responsibility by putting medical decision making back in the hands of provider groups, along with fiscal responsibility for the viability of the plan for which they work.

A comprehensive benefit package was laid out to be subject to fine tuning and modification over time by the National Health Board (*Health Security*, 1993). Its description took up 92 pages in the text of the CHP Bill submitted to Congress. It included virtually all inpatient, outpatient, short- and long-term, institutional and home-based, preventive, diagnostic, treatment, rehabilitative, and follow-up services.

Each person would have been able to choose from among three types of coverage (*Health Security*, 1993): an HMO with no deductible and a copayment of no more than $10.00 for each doctor visit; a PPO, with no deductible and a $10.00 copayment if the patient were to use network providers, deductibles and higher copayments for the use of physicians outside the PPO (which would be permitted); and a fee-for-service system (like the managed care point-of-service option) allowing completely free choice of doctor, with significant deductibles and copayments. (Under the latter option there would be a fee schedule for the physicians, and no balance billing would be allowed.) For most businesses, large and small, participation would have been mandated, a major bone of contention. Because employers would have no say in plan choice by their employees, change from plan to plan would be only at the individual's option (unless a plan went out of business). Coverage would be portable from job to job and from job to no job.

Finally, the CHP would have linked payment and planning, under public rather than private control, the *desideratum* so eloquently set forth by Dr. Rashi Fein (see chapter 7). That would have enabled (although not guaranteed) significant health care delivery system (HCDS) reform. This was, perhaps, what the opponents of the CHP were most afraid of.

The Opposition

Republican political guru William Kristol was an early leader of the opposition to the CHP. In the first of the then soon-to-be-famous "Kristol Memos" (1993), he said:

> The Clinton proposal is a serious *political* threat to the Republican Party. Republicans must therefore clearly understand the political strategy implicit in the Clinton plan—and then adopt an aggressive and uncompromising counterstrategy designed to delegitimize the proposal and defeat its partisan purpose.

On the provider side, most of the medical, hospital, and insurance/managed care industry groups were arrayed against it, for a variety of reasons, ranging from an antagonism to "government regulation" to a concern with potential limitations on profit-making ability. On the public side, the "single-payer" forces were also arrayed against it, at least its leadership was (Navarro, 1994). They felt that it didn't go far enough, that it left too many players in Big Health Care in place. They assumed that if the CHP was defeated, their approach would next be on center stage of the health care agenda. Unfortunately, history seems to have proved them wrong.

Finally, "Big Business," represented by such groups as the U.S. Chamber of Commerce and the National Association of Manufacturers, had originally been thought to be supporters of the CHP, at least by the Clinton people. They were wrong. Industry groups, by and large, eventually came out in opposition to the CHP (Hacker, 1996). Also a factor in the defeat of the CHP was the fact that although the CHP appeared to be well thought out and adapted to the American political and HCDS realities (as one observer said, "product development was good") there was no comprehensive marketing plan prepared by the forces supporting it (Hacker, 1996). Thus, under a lengthy and expensive onslaught, the CHP went down to defeat in the summer of 1994 (Skocpol, 1995).

LOOKING AHEAD

Many of the major problems in the U.S. health care delivery system are national ones. They require national solutions. That does not necessarily mean a federally run national health service. That ''solution'' would probably work poorly in this country for many reasons. But it does mean national principles and guidelines, national programs for change.

To stem the tide of rising medical and hospital costs, some influential policy groups such as the Heritage Foundation (1989) have placed their major emphasis on the promotion of ''competition'' in the health care delivery system, to be stimulated by ''consumer/patient choice.'' For competition to be effective in lowering prices and improving quality, however, the consumer must have some reasonable knowledge of what he/she is buying. Furthermore, he/she must make the most of the purchases.

In health care, however, just the opposite is true. Most consumers know virtually nothing about what they are buying and could care less, just as long as they get better. Further, it is in any case the sellers (that is, the health care providers), not the consumers, who make the majority of the decisions about what shall be purchased on behalf of which consumers at what price.

It is popular in some circles to say that NHI is too expensive, that the nation cannot afford it. According to proponents of the comprehensive plans the truth is just the opposite. They say that with the skyrocketing costs, questionable quality, increases in preventable death in certain segments of the population (*MVSR*, 1990; Rosenthal, 1990; E. Schwartz et al., 1990), and massive misallocation of resources that occur under the present voluntary, ''free'' system (Woolhandler & Himmelstein, 1991), the nation cannot afford *not* to have it.

It must be recognized, however, that any NHI plan that does not tackle the *causes* of the problems head on, any plan that just pays in a different way for the system we now have, will in the long run likely make things worse, not better. We must not just pay differently for things; we must pay for different things. But making rational, planned, national change in the U.S. health care delivery system is very difficult, as history has taught us again and again, most recently in the battle over the Clinton Health Plan in the mid-1990s.

The several provider groupings are very powerful. Traditionally, the two most powerful were the physicians and the hospitals. In the past, major changes in the system have taken place only when the physicians and/or the hospitals wanted or needed those changes. Examples include the reinstitution of medical licensing laws and the reduction in the number of medical schools in the late 19th and early 20th centuries, and the development of voluntary hospital insurance during the Great Depression.

NHI might finally come when one or the other or both of those groups want it or need it. The private hospitals might want it as an increasing number of them go bankrupt in the face of uncontrolled cost increases and declining occupancy rates, as happened in Great Britain just before the enactment of their National Health Service in 1946. The physicians might want it when their numbers are so large that they will no longer be able to sell all the product they can collectively produce, as they can now. If this were to happen while a majority of them were still private entrepreneurs, the competition would be chaotic (Consumer Commission, 1978). The shelter of a secure, if somewhat smaller income might be sought in salaried service.

In the mid-1990s, however, the situation was complicated by the emerging power of the insurance industry coupled with the sometimes separate, sometimes intertwined power of the for-profit managed care sector. Sometimes those interests coincide with those of the traditional holders of power, as they did in the fight over the CHP. That is not to say that they might not diverge in the future, however.

Proposals for solutions abound, as noted above. None of them are perfect in anyone's eyes. Nevertheless, some have more potential for solving the major problems than do others. Those with the most potential have one key characteristic in common: proactive, not reactive, planning, linked to financing. One must bear in mind the question Henrik Blum asked in 1983, however: "Can there be meaningful health planning [in the United States] when so little else is planned?"

Finally, one can ask, if there is no planning, no system, no national program, what will happen? Some predict major catastrophe and crisis. But in spite of predictions of impending doom going back 25 years and more (see chapter 1), no national catastrophe has occurred (although millions of individuals have been hard done by). The system just keeps barreling along, getting ever-more expensive, and showing major defects in both the quality and the quantity of service provided. Will there indeed be a crisis? Will there be a catastrophe? Or will we just continue to experience more of the same? The outcome of this drama is one that no one can predict.

REFERENCES

AMA (American Medical Association). *Health access America*. Chicago, IL: Author, March 1990.

Anderson, O. W. *The uneasy equilibrium: Private and public financing of health services in the United States, 1875–1965*. New Haven, CT: College and University Press, 1968.

Blum, H. L. [Review of *Health planning: Lessons for the future*, by Bonnie Lefkowitz.] *Inquiry, 20,* 390, 1983.

Burns, E. M. Health insurance: Not if, or when, but what kind? *American Journal of Public Health, 61,* 2164, 1971.

Burrow, J. G. *AMA: Voice of American medicine*. Baltimore: Johns Hopkins University Press, 1963.

Burrow, J. G. *Organized medicine in the progressive era*. Baltimore, MD: Johns Hopkins University Press, 1977.

Canada's threatened healthcare system. *The Lancet, 345,* 1995.

Cavalier, K. *National health insurance*. Washington DC: Congressional Research Service, Library of Congress, 1979.

Committee on the Costs of Medical Care. *Medical care for the American people*. Washington, DC: USDHEW, 1970. (Original work published 1932.)

Committee on Finance, United States Senate. *Medicare and Medicaid: Problems, issues and alternatives*. Washington, DC: U.S.G.P.O., 1970.

Committee on Finance, United States Senate. *Comparison of major features of health insurance proposals*. Washington, DC: U.S.G.P.O., 1979.

Committee on Labor and Human Resources. *Background information on S. 1265, The Minimum Health Benefits for All Workers Act of 1988*. Washington, DC: US Senate Committee on Labor and Human Resources, April 29, 1988.

Committee on Medical Care Teaching of the Association of Teachers of Preventive Medicine. *Readings in medical care*. Chapel Hill, NC: University of North Carolina Press, 1958a. (Reprinted from Boas, F. P. *Why do we need national health insurance?* Society for Ethical Culture, 1945.)

Committee on Medical Care Teaching of the Association of Teachers of Preventive Medicine. *Readings in Medical Care*. Chapel Hill, NC: University of North Carolina Press, 1958b. (Reprinted from McKittrick, L. S. Medical care for the American people: Is compulsory health insurance the solution? *New England Journal of Medicine, 240,* 998, 1949.)

Committee on Medical Care Teaching. *Readings in Medical Care*. Chapel Hill, NC: University of North Carolina Press, 1958c, p. 629. (Reprinted from Truman, H. S. *Message from the President of the United States*, 79th Congress, 1st Session. Washington, DC: U.S.G.P.O., 1945.)

Committee for National Health Insurance. *The health security partnership*. Washington, DC: Committee for National Health Insurance, 1989.

Committee on Ways and Means, House of Representatives. *National health insurance resource book*. Washington, DC: U.S.G.P.O., 1974.

Consumer Commission on the Accreditation of Health Services. National health service V: Building a medical staff. *Consumer Health Perspectives, 5*(3), 1, 1978.

Davis, K. *National health insurance: Benefits, costs, and consequences*. Washington, DC: Brookings Institution, 1975.

The delivery challenges posed by Canada: A bilateral view. *Hospitals*, November 5, 1990, p. 58.

Douglas-Wilson, I., & McLachlan, G. *Health service prospects: An international survey*. Boston: Little, Brown, 1973.

Eilers, R. D. National health insurance: What kind and how much? Parts 1 and 2. *New England Journal of Medicine, 284,* 881, 945, 1971.

Evans, R. G. et al. Controlling health expenditures—The Canadian reality. *New England Journal of Medicine, 320,* 571, 1989.

Falk, I. S. Medical care in the USA, 1932–1972. Problems, proposals and programs from the Committee on the Costs of Medical Care to the Committee for National Health Insurance. *Health and Society, 51,* 1, 1973.

Falk, I. S. Proposals for national health insurance in the USA: Origins and evolution, and some perceptions for the future. *Health and Society*, Spring 1977, p. 161.

Freeland, R. M. *The Truman doctrine and the origins of McCarthyism*. New York: Knopf, 1975.

Freudenheim, M. Health industry is changing itself ahead of reform. *New York Times*, June 27, 1994, p. A1.

Friedman, E. Medicaid. Part 1. *Hospitals, 51,* August 16, 1977, p. 51; Part 2. *Hospitals, 51,* September 1, 1977, p. 59; Part 3. *Hospitals, 51,* September 16, 1977, p. 73; Part 4. *Hospitals, 51,* October 1, 1977, p. 61; Part 5. *Hospitals, 51,* November 1, 1977, p. 77.

Fry, J., & Farndale, W. A. J. (Eds.). *International medical care*. Oxford, England: MTP, 1972.

Fuchs, V. R., & Hahn, J. S. How does Canada do it? *New England Journal of Medicine, 323,* 884, 1990.

GAO (General Accounting Office). *Canadian health insurance: Lessons for the United States*. Washington, DC: GAO/HRD-91-90, June 1991.

GAO (General Accounting Office). *Canadian health insurance: Estimating cost and savings for the United States*. Washington, DC: GAO/HRD-92-83, April 1992.

Glaser, W. A. *Health insurance bargaining*. New York: Gardner Press, 1978.

Goodman, W. E. Canada's health-care system: You get what you pay for. *Private Practice*, October, 1989, p. 11.

Grumbach, K. et al. Liberal benefits, conservative spending: The physicians for a national health program proposal. *Journal of the American Medical Association, 265,* 2549, 1991.

Hacker, J. S. National health care reform: An idea whose time came and went. *Journal of Health Politics, Policy and Law, 21,* 647, Winter 1996.

Harris, R. Annals of legislation: Medicare. *The New Yorker*, July 2, July 9, July 16, July 23, 1966.

Health Security: The President's Report to the American People. Washington, DC: The Domestic Policy Council, The White House, October 1993.

Heritage Foundation. *Critical issues: A national health system for America.* Washington, DC: Heritage Foundation, 1989.

Himmelstein, D. U., & Woolhandler, S. A national health program for the United States. *New England Journal of Medicine, 320,* 102, 1989.

Igelhart, J. Canada's health care system. Parts 1, 2, 3, *New England Journal of Medicine, 315,* 202, 778, 1623, 1986.

Igelhart, J. Canada's health care system faces it's problems. *New England Journal of Medicine, 322,* 562, 1990.

IOM (Institute of Medicine, Committee on Health Planning Goals and Standards). *Health planning in the United States: Selected policy issues.* Washington, DC: National Academy Press, 1981.

Insurance plan stresses reform, prevention. *The Nation's Health*, March 1990, p. 1.

Jonas, S. Issues in national health insurance in the United States of America. *The Lancet*, July 20, 1974, p. 143.

Jonas, S. *Quality-control of ambulatory care.* New York: Springer Publishing Co., 1977.

Jonas, S. National health insurance. In S. Jonas (Ed.), *Health care delivery in the United States* (2nd ed.). New York: Springer Publishing Co., 1981a.

Jonas, S. Planning for national health insurance by objective: The contract mechanism. In R. Straetz (Ed.), *Critical perspectives and issues in health policy.* Lexington, MA: Lexington Books, 1981b.

Jonas, S. The personal health care system. *New York State Journal of Medicine, 84,* 187, 1984.

Kimble, C. Special report: Comparing the Carter and Kennedy national health insurance bills. *Washington Report on Medicine and Health.* November, 1979.

Kristol, W. Defeating President Clinton's health care proposal. Washington, DC: Project for the Republican Future (memo), December 2, 1993.

Linton, A. L. The Canadian health care system: A Canadian physician's perspective. *New England Journal of Medicine, 322,* 197, 1990.

Lynch, M. J., & Raphael, S. S. *Medicine and the state.* Springfield, IL: Charles C Thomas, 1963.

Lyons, S. A. The birth of the Canadian health care system. *PNHP Newsletter*, July 1996.

McMahon, J. A. *Statement of the American Hospital Association on national health insurance before the Health Subcommittee of the House Committee on Ways and Means.* November 10, 1975. Washington, DC: American Hospital Association.

MVSR (*Monthly Vital Statistics Report*). Advance report of final mortality statistics, 1988. *39*(7), (Suppl.), November 28, 1990.

National Association of Manufacturers. *Meeting the health care crisis*. Washington, DC: 1989.

National Leadership Commission on Health Care. *For the health of a nation: A shared responsibility*. Ann Arbor, MI: Health Administration Press Perspectives, 1989.

Navarro, V. The need to mobilize support for the Wellstone-McDermott-Conyers single-payer proposal. *American Journal of Public Health, 84,* 178, 1994.

New York Academy of Medicine. Toward a national health program. *Bulletin of New York Academy of Medicine, 48,* January 1972.

Nolan, N. Bitter medicine. *In These Times*, January 20, 1997, p. 16.

Oil, Chemical and Atomic Workers. *National Health Care: Pass it On!* Lakewood, CO: OCAW, 1989.

Redlener, I. *Presentation, Rockland County Democratic Forum*. New York: November 10, 1993.

Roemer, M. I. I.S. Falk, the Committee on the Costs of Medical Care, and the drive for national health insurance. *American Journal of Public Health, 75,* 841, 1985.

Roemer, M. I. *National health systems of the world, volume one, the countries*. New York: Oxford University Press, 1991.

Rosenthal, E. Health problems of the inner city poor reach crisis point. *New York Times*, December 24, 1990, p. A1.

Schwartz, E. et al. Black/white comparisons of deaths preventable by medical intervention: United States and the District of Columbia 1980–86. *International Journal of Epidemiology, 19,* 591, 1990.

Schwartz, H. *The case for American medicine: A realistic look at our health care system*. New York: David McKay, 1972.

Sigerist, H. E. *On the sociology of medicine*. M. I. Roemer, (Ed.). New York: MD Publications, 1960.

Skocpol, T. The rise and resounding demise of the Clinton Health Plan. *Health Affairs, 14,* 61, 1995.

Stark, Kennedy to Propose Health Reforms. *Washington Report on Medicine and Health*, June 17, 1985.

Stevens, R. *American medicine and the public interest*. New Haven, CT: Yale University Press, 1971.

U.S. Bipartisan Commission on Comprehensive Health Care. *A call for action*. Washington, DC: U.S.G.P.O., September 1990.

Woolhandler, S., & Himmelstein, D. U. A national health program: Northern light at the end of the tunnel. *Journal of the American Medical Association, 262,* 2136, 1989a.

Woolhandler, S., & Himmelstein, D. U. Resolving the cost/access conflict. *Journal of General Internal Medicine, 4,* 54, 1989b.

Woolhandler, S., & Himmelstein, D. U. The deteriorating administrative efficiency of the U.S. health care system. *The New England Journal of Medicine, 324,* 1253, 1991.

Appendix I

List of Selected Critical Reports/Analyses of the U.S Health Care Delivery System 1927–1990

Business Week, ''The $60-Billion Crisis over Medical Care.'' Special reprint, January 17, 1970.

Citizen's Board of Inquiry into Health Services for Americans, *Heal Yourself* (Report). Washington, D.C.: Citizen's Board of Inquiry into Health Services, for Americans, 1971.

Committee for National Health Insurance, *The Health Security Partnership.* Washington, DC: 1989.

Ehrenreich, B., & Ehrenreich, J., *The American Health Empire: Power, Profits, and Politics*, New York: Vintage Books, 1971.

Harper's Magazine, ''The Crisis in American Medicine.'' October 1960, p. 123.

Healthline, ''American Health Care: A System in Crisis.'' October 1983, p. 7.

Health Task Force of the Urban Coalition, *Rx for Action* (Report). Washington, D.C.: 1969.

Jonas, S., *Medical Mystery: The Training of Doctors in the United States.* New York: W. W. Norton, 1979.

Kennedy, E. M., *In Critical Condition.* New York: Simon and Schuster, 1972.

Knowles, J. H. (Ed.), *Doing Better and Feeling Worse.* New York: W. W. Norton, 1977.

Moskin, J. R., ''The Challenge to Our Doctors.'' *Look*, November 3, 1964, p. 26.

National Commission on Community Health Services, *Health Is a Community Affair*. Cambridge, MA: Harvard University Press. 1966.

National Leadership Commission on Health Care, *For the Health of a Nation: A Shared Responsibility*, Ann Arbor, MI: Health Administration Press Perspectives, 1989.

Pepper Commission, *A Call for Action*, Executive Summary. Washington, DC: US Government Printing Office, September, 1990.

Ribicoff, A., with Danaceau, P., *The American Medical Machine*. New York: Saturday Review Press, 1972.

Schorr, D., *Don't Get Sick in America*. Nashville, Tenn.: Aurora Publishers, 1970.

Silver, G. A., *A Spy in the House of Medicine*. Germantown, MD: Aspen Systems Corporation, 1976.

Somers, A. R., & Somers, H. M., *Health and Health Care*. Germantown, MD: Aspen Systems Corporation, 1977.

U.S. Bipartisan Commission on Comprehensive Health Care, *A Call for Action*. Washington, DC: USGPO, September, 1990.

Further, in a review of the Ehrenreich & Ehrenreich book, *The American Health Empire: Power, Profits, and Politics* (cited above), that appeared in the *International Journal of Health Services*, (2, 119, 1972), Dr. Milton Roemer listed a series of other reports going back many years. He said (p. 119):

> Every few years, more recently in the last decade, there appears a book analyzing the serious defects of health care in America. In 1927, Harry H. Moore produced *American Medicine and the People's Health*, in the 1930's were the magnificent 27 volumes of the Committee on the Costs of Medical Care, in 1939 there was James Rorty's *American Medicine Mobilizes*, and in 1940 Hugh Cabot's *The Patient Dilemma*. After World War II, Carl Malmberg wrote *140 Million Patients* in 1947, Michael Davis wrote *Medical Care for Tomorrow* in 1955, and Richard Carter wrote *The Doctor Business* in 1958. In 1965 there was Selig Greenberg's excellent *The Troubled Calling: Crisis in the Medical Establishment*. The year after Medicare, 1966, saw two critical outputs: *The American Health Scandal* by Raul Tunley and *The Doctors* by Martin L. Gross. In 1967 there was Fred J. Cook's *Plot Against the Patient* and in 1970 Ed Cray's *In Failing Health*.

Appendix II

A Guide to Sources of Data

INTRODUCTION

This Appendix is a guide to the principal sources of health and health services data for the United States, as of 1997. It contains descriptions of those sources, indicates how frequently each is published, lists the categories of data and other information they contain, and gives the address of the publisher of each and other ordering information as indicated.

There are two comprehensive guides to sources of data that are published annually. The first appears in *Health, United States* (see item # 7, below; the most recent edition as of this writing is for 1995, published in May, 1996 [DHHS Pub. No. (PHS) 96-1232]). Its Appendix I contains very useful, detailed descriptions of all the common health data sources published by the several branches of the Federal government, the United Nations, and private agencies ranging from the American Medical Association to the National League for Nursing, usually including addresses.

The second appears in the *Statistical Abstract of the United States* (see item # 1, below; the most recent edition as of this writing is for 1996, published in September, 1996). Appendix I contains an extensive listing of sources of health data (as well as the sources of all other data appearing in the *Statistical Abstract*). Appendix III of that publication presents brief descriptions of, and analyses of the limitations of, the major sources of data listed in Appendix I.

Almost all Federal sources of data are available for purchase through the United Government Printing Office (USGPO or GPO, for short), Superintendent of Documents, P.O. Box 371954, Pittsburgh, PA 15250-7954, tel. (202) 512-1800, FAX (202) 512-2250. There are local USGPO bookstores and phone ordering centers located in major cities around the

United States. They are listed in the Federal government section of the blue pages of the respective local telephone directories under ''Government Printing Office.''

Also, the *AHA Guide*, published annually by the American Hospital Association (see item # 10, below), in its Part C lists the major national, international, U.S. government, state and local government, and private ''Health Organizations, Agencies, and Providers'' with addresses and telephone numbers. Health and health care data can be obtained from many of them.

PRINCIPAL SOURCES OF HEALTH AND HEALTH CARE DATA

1. *Statistical Abstract of the United States.* Published annually by the Bureau of the Census, U.S. Department of Commerce, Washington, DC 20233, the *Statistical Abstract* contains a vast collection of tables reporting information and data collected by many different government (and in certain cases nongovernment) agencies. They are accumulated under the following headings: Population; Vital Statistics; Health and Nutrition; Education; Law Enforcement, Courts, and Prisons; Geography and Environment; Parks, Recreation, and Travel; Elections; State and Local Government Finances and Employment; Federal Government Finances and Employment; National Defense and Veterans' Affairs; Social Insurance and Human Services; Social Insurance and Human Services; Labor Force, Employment, and Earnings; Income, Expenditures, and Wealth; Prices; Banking, Finance, and Insurance; Business Enterprise; Communications; Energy; Science; Transportation—Land; Transportation—Air and Water; Agriculture; Natural Resources; Construction and Housing; Manufactures; Domestic Trade and Services; Foreign Commerce and Aid; Outlying Areas [under the Jurisdiction of the United States]; Comparative International Statistics; and Industrial Outlook. There are health and health services data of varying kinds reported in many of these categories, although the principal ones are of course found under Population, Vital Statistics, and Health and Nutrition.

2. *U.S. Census of Population.* As noted above, the Bureau of the Census is part of the U.S. Department of Commerce. The United States Constitution requires that a census be taken every 10 years, at the beginning of each decade. The original purpose of the census was to apportion seats in the House of Representatives, thus also distributing the seats in the Electoral College which was to choose the President. In modern times, in addition to the simple counts, a great deal of demographic data is collected by the Census Bureau. Many reports on the decennial censuses

as well as interim special counts are published by the Census Bureau (see item # 3, below). But a good place to begin is in Section 1 of the *Statistical Abstract*. Considerably more detailed information is published periodically in hardcover compendia of decennial national census data. Also available are special analyses for a wide variety of geographical subdivisions of the country. Census Bureau publications may be ordered from the USGPO which offers for sale a comprehensive *Census Catalog and Guide*. Many Census Bureau products are also available through a desktop computer on-line service called CENDATA, as well as in the Compact Disc:Read Only Memory (CD:ROM) format. Electronic product orders may be sent to the U.S. Department of Commerce, Bureau of the Census, P.O. Box 277943, Atlanta, GA 30384-7943, tel. (301) 457-4100, FAX (301) 457-3842.

3. *Current Population Reports*. In addition to reports from the decennial censuses, the Census Bureau publishes seven series of reports on a continuing basis, called "Current Population Reports." These include estimates, projections, sample counts, and special studies of selected segments of the population. The seven series each have a "P" number. They are: P-20, Population Characteristics; P-23, Special Studies; P-25, Population Estimates and Projections; P-26, Local Population Estimates; P-28, Special Censuses; P-60, Consumer Income; P-70, Household Economic Studies. Catalogs and information on the content of each series are available directly from the Bureau of the Census, U.S. Department of Commerce, Washington, D.C., 20233. Publications may be ordered through the USGPO.

4. *Monthly Vital Statistics Report (MVSR)*. MVSR is published by the National Center for Health Statistics (NCHS), Centers for Disease Control and Prevention (CDCP), Public Health Service (PHS), U.S. Department of Health and Human Services (USDHHS), 6525 Belcrest Road, Hyattsville, MD 20782, telephone (301) 436-8500. The NCHS periodically publishes catalogs of its various publications and electronic data products, available free. The *MVSR* has several sections. "Provisional Data," published monthly, contain the most recent data for the traditional "vital statistics"—births, marriages, divorces, and deaths. There is a series of "Supplements" that appear on a semi-regular basis, containing "Advance Reports" of the "Final Data" for the annually collected vital statistics. There are also reports entitled "Advance Data." They present regularly collected "Vital and Health Statistics" on the health care delivery system from, for example, the "National Home and Hospice Care Survey," the "National Hospital Ambulatory Medical Care Survey," and the "National Hospital Discharge Survey," as well as the results of special studies and

technical information on methodology. All MVSR reports may be obtained by annual subscription, through the USGPO.

5. *Vital Statistics of the United States.* These are the full, highly detailed annual reports on vital statistics from the NCHS, the summary versions of which are published in the Supplements of the *MVSR.*

6. *Vital and Health Statistics.* These publications of the NCHS, distinct from the "Vital Statistics" reports described in items 4 and 5 above, appear at irregular intervals. As of 1997, there were 14 series, not numbered consecutively. Most of them report data from ongoing studies and surveys that the NCHS has carried out. The publication of some data shifts periodically between *Vital and Health Statistics* and *Monthly Vital Statistics Report.* The 14 series of *Vital and Health Statistics* are as follows: Series 1, Programs and Collection Procedures; Series 2, Data Evaluation and Methods Research; Series 3, Analytical and Epidemiological Studies; Series 4, Documents and Committee Reports; Series 5, International Vital and Health Statistics Reports; Series 6, Cognition and Survey Measurement; Series 10, Data from the Health Interview Survey; Series 11, Data from the National Health Examination Survey, the National Health and Nutrition Examination Surveys, and the Hispanic Health and Nutrition Examination Survey; Series 13, Data on Health Resources Utilization; Series 16, Compilations of Advance Data from Vital and Health Statistics; Series 20, Data on Mortality; Series 21, Data on Natality, Marriage, and Divorce; Series 24, Compilations of Data on Natality, Mortality, Marriage, Divorce, and Induced Terminations of Pregnancy.

7. *Health, United States.* This is published annually by the NCHS/CDCP, and available for purchase from the USGPO. A wide variety of health and health care delivery system data are presented, under the following categories: population, fertility and natality, mortality, determinants of health, utilization of health resources, health care resources, and health care expenditures. It also contains a useful appendix, Sources and Limitations of Data, as well as a Glossary. It is a boon to students and researchers in health care delivery because it provides one-stop shopping for most important health and health care data.

8. *Morbidity and Mortality Weekly Report (MMWR).* This is a regular publication of the Centers for Disease Control and Prevention of the PHS, USDHHS. It is available on an annual subscription basis from the USGPO. However, following a large subscription price increase in 1982, *MMWR,* in the public domain, has been photocopied and circulated at cost by several organizations, including the Massachusetts Medical Society, P.O. Box 9120, Waltham, MA 02254-9120. In the past, MMWR has been concerned primarily with communicable disease reporting. These reports are still included, as of 1997 for AIDS, chlamydia, *Escherichia coli,*

gonorrhea, viral hepatitis, Legionellosis, Lyme disease, malaria, *H. influenzae* (invasive), measles, meningococcal disease, mumps, pertussis, and rubella, primary and secondary syphilis, tuberculosis, and animal rabies. MMWR also reports deaths in 122 U.S. cities on a weekly basis. In the late 1990s, equally or perhaps more important, each week MMWR presents brief reports on special studies of such diverse health topics as: alcohol consumption among pregnant and childbearing-aged women, human rabies, progress towards global poliomyelitis eradication, rubella and congenital rubella syndrome in the U.S., adult blood lead epidemiology and surveillance, Clean Air Month, urban community intervention to prevent Halloween arson, sports-related recurrent brain injuries, a tobacco tax initiative in Oregon, and prevalence of cigarette smoking among secondary school students in Budapest, Hungary. MMWR also periodically publishes ''Recommendations and Reports'' of various governmental and nongovernmental health agencies and organizations, and the results of ''CDC Surveillance Summaries.''

9. *Health Care Financing Review*. This is a quarterly publication of the Health Care Financing Administration (HCFA), USDHHS, Office of Research and Demonstrations, 1-A-9 Oak Meadows Building, 7500 Security Boulevard, C3-11-07, Baltimore, MD 21244-1850. telephone (410) 786-6572. It is available by subscription through the USGPO. It annually publishes the official reports, ''National Health Expenditures'' and ''Health Care Indicators.'' It also publishes an extensive and wide-ranging series of academic articles, reports, and studies, with an emphasis on Medicare/Medicaid (for which HCFA is directly responsible), but also covering ''a broad range of health care financing and delivery issues.''

10. *American Hospital Association Guide to the Health Care Field*. This is a two-part publication of the American Hospital Association, One North Franklin, Chicago, Illinois 60606-3401, publication ordering telephone (800) AHA-2626, available for purchase from the AHA. The first part, the *AHA Guide*, as of the late 1990s is published biennially. It contains a listing of almost every hospital in the United States by location and gives basic data on size, type, ownership, and facilities, a listing and brief description of the Integrated Health Care Delivery Networks, the Multi-hospital Health Care Systems, and information on the AHA itself, as well as the comprehensive lists of health and health care organizations referred to in the introductory section of the Appendix, above. The second part, *AHA Hospital Statistics*, as of the mid-1990s is also published biennially. It contains a great deal of summary descriptive, utilization, and financial data on U.S. hospitals, presented in many different cross-tabulations. Some of the data are presented historically as well. The two parts

together contain the most detailed data available on hospitals in the United States.

11. *Center for Health Policy Research of the American Medical Association.* The Center, located in AMA National Headquarters, 515 North State Street, Chicago, Illinois 60610, ordering telephone number (800) 621-8335 produces a variety of useful data on the physician work force and related subjects. As of 1997, titles appearing on a regular basis included: "Socioeconomic Characteristics of Medical Practice," "Physician Marketplace Statistics," "U.S. Medical Licensure Statistics and Current Licensure Requirements," "Physician Characteristics and Distribution in the U.S.," and "Medical Groups in the U.S."

Index

Access to health care, US, 2
Acute-care hospitals, 7
Aetna, 92
African Americans
 infant mortality rate, 5
 life expectancy, 4, 105
 medical school admissions, 33
 patient visits, 68
Age adjusted death rates, 5
Agency for Health Care Policy and Research, 111, 113
Agriculture Department, 13, 110, 115
AHA Guide to the Health Care Field, The, 46
Aid to Families with Dependent Children (AFDC), 97
AIDS control program, 111
Allopathic medical schools, 32
Alzheimer's disease, 5
Ambulance medical services, 74, 75
Ambulatory care, 7, 29, 67–69. *See also* Primary care
Ambulatory services, outside hospital, 74
American Association for Labor Legislation, 167
American Cancer Society, 14, 109
American College of Preventive Medicine, 14
American Federation of Labor, 167
American Heart Association, 13–14, 109
American Hospital Association (AHA), 7, 46, 134
 on national health insurance, 171
American Medical Association (AMA), 14, 32, 147
 on national health insurance, 167–168, 169, 170, 171, 176
 opposition to regionalization, 135
 registered care technician (RCT), 36–37
American Medical Athletics Association, 14
American Nurses Association (ANA), 14
 definition of nursing, 34
American Osteopathic Association, 32
American Public Health Association, 176
"Ameriplan," 174
Arthritis, 5
Asian, medical school admissions, 33
Association of American Medical Colleges, 32
Association of State and Territorial Health Officials (ASTHO), 117
Asthma and hay fever, 5
Atherosclerosis, 5
Audiologists, 26, 41
Australia, infant mortality rate, 4
Average daily census, 48, 49

"i" indicates an illustration; "t" indicates a table; "fn" indicates a footnote

Basic Health Planning Methods (Spiegel and Hyman), 124
"Basic six," 117
Bellevue Hospital (NY), 46
Biomedical research, purpose of, 8
Bipartisan Commission on Comprehensive Health Care, 176
Blood infection, leading cause of death, 5
Blue Cross/Blue Shield, private insurance, 9, 92, 160
"Bodily tissue," 55
British Commonwealth, national health insurance, 167

California, mature managed care market, 145
Canada
  GDP expended on health care, 85
  infant mortality rate, 4
  national health insurance program, 176–178
  national health system, four principles, 176, 177
Cancer, 5, 135
Capitation, 9–10, 99, 100
Cardiorespiratory therapists, 26
Causes of disease, leading, 5
Center for Disease Control and Prevention (CDCP), 111, 112, 117
Center for Nursing, nurse extender, 37
Child health, public health agencies, 75
Children, patient visits, 68, 73
Chiropractors, 26
Clinical psychology, hospital division, 55
"Clinical-practice plan," 71
Clinics, groups of, 71
Clinton Health Plan. *See* Health Security Act of 1993
Coinsurance, 92–93
Commission on Hospital Care, 134
Commission on Public-General Hospitals, AHA, 56
Committee on Economic Security, 168
Committee on Health Planning Goals and Standards, 139, 175
Committee on National Health Insurance, 176
Committee on the Costs of Medical Care (CCMC), 19, 21, 65, 134, 159, 168
Committee on the Future of Public Health, 105, 119
Commodities, health care, 6, 7–8, 14, 84
Communicable Disease Center, 111
Community Health Centers (CHCs), 68, 77–78. *See also* Neighborhood Health Community hospital
Community hospital, 7, 47, 48t, 49
  bed:population ratio, 50
Community Mental Health Centers, 68
Community-oriented primary care, elements of, 72–73
Community-Oriented Primary Care (COPC) model, 77
"Comprehensive care medicine," 63–64. *See also* Primary care
Comprehensive diagnostic centers, 74
Computerized axial tomography (CAT) scanning, 53
Congressional Research Service, on national health insurance, 172, 173
Consumer Report, on managed care, 144, 145
Corporate profits, from U.S. health care services, 2
Council on Graduate Medical Education (COGME), sixth report, 31
"Critical care," 53

Dawson Report, 159
Death, leading causes of, 5
Deductibles, 92
Defense Department, 98, 110, 115
Demographic data, 130
Denmark, national health care system, 4–5
Dentists, 9, 25
Diabetes mellitus, leading cause of death, 5

Diagnosis
home health care, 80
hospice care, 80
most frequent emergency room, 73
most frequent outpatient, 70
most frequent primary care, 69
"Diagnosis-Related Group (DRG)," 96
Dietary patterns, 5
Dieticians, 25
Distribution of health care services, United States, 2
Doctor-nurse game, 39
"Domiciliares," 114
"Drug-Free America," 126
Drug use, 5
"Drug War," 126

Elderly
home health care, 80
hospitalization of, 51
patient visits, 68, 70, 73
Elizabethan Poor Laws, 105
Emergency departments (EDs), 69. *See also* Emergency services
Emergency medical services, 75
in hospitals, 73–74
nonhospital, 74
Employee health services, 15
Environmental Protection Administration (EPA), 13, 110, 116
Europe, national health insurance, 167
Evaluations, of health programs, 133
Exclusive provider organization (EPO), 156
Executive branch, government role in health care, 108
Extra charges, 93

Family planning, public health agencies, 76
Federal government
employment of physicians, 27
as health care provider, 109, 110–116
Federal hospital, 47, 48t
Fee-for service, 2, 9, 28, 97, 99, 148, 177
Fee-for-service system, Health Security Act, 180
Financing, health care, 6, 8–9, 84, 109–110
Firearms, 5
Food and Drug Administration, 111, 112
Food Stamp program, 115
Fortune Magazine, on medical costs, 19
"Foundation for Medical Care," 151
14th Amendment, 107, 108
Functional program goals, 128

"Gatekeeper," 29, 64, 73
General hospital, 47, 56
General practitioners
in Great Britain, 29
in United States, 68
Germany, national insurance program, 166–167
Ghetto medicine, 174
Global budgeting, payment mode, 99, 100
Goals, of health planning, 125, 132
Goshen Emergency Hospital (NY), 70
Government, as funding source, 88, 93, 94t–95t, 96–98
Great Britain, health care system, 29, 65
Gross domestic product (GDP), percent expended on health care, 85
Group medical practice, 146–151
prepaid, 148–151
private, 147–148
Group model, 150, 154
HMOs, 68
Guide to Clinical Preventive Services, The, 113

Health and Human Resources (DHHS), Department of, 13, 110–113
Health care
costs, methods of payment, 9
data, 130
delivery system, 6–10, 18–19, 67, 84, 129
expenditures for, 94t–95t, 98–99

Health care *(continued)*
expenditures on, 84–85, 86t–87t
funding sources, 88, 89i, 90t–91t, 92–98
payments, modes of, 99–100
planning, defined, 10, 139
Health Care Alliances, 179, 180
Health Care Corporation, 174
Health care system
administration of, 11–12
major problems of, 146
program evaluation, 11
regulation of, 11
Health insurance, health service fundor, 88
Health Insurance Plan (HIP), 149
Health Maintenance Organization (HMO), 144, 145, 153, 152, 154–155
Health measurements, 130–131
Health Net, 160
Health planning, 123 fn 1, 123–129
Health professional organizations, 14
Health Resources and Services Administration, 111
Health risk factors, 131
Health Security Act of 1993, 3, 20, 96–97, 106, 165, 178, 179–180, 181
Health services
delivery of, 16–18
goals, federal, 138
programs, 12
special populations, 17
usage, measurement, 131
Health statistics, 117
Health status goals, federal, 138
Health Systems Agency (HSA), roles and functions, 137–138
Health: United States, 47
Healthy People 2000: Midcourse Review and 1995 Revisions, 113, 138
Healthy People 2000: National Health Promotion and Disease Prevention Objectives, 113, 138
Heart disease, 5, 135
Henricopolis, 46
Heritage Foundation, 176, 182
Hill-Burton Act. *See* Hospital Survey and Construction Act
Home care
and hospice, 80
hospital division, 55
Hospital(s)
admissions, physicians role in, 3
bed formula, 50
beds, distribution and supply, 50
decline in, 51, 56
divisions, 52, 55
emergency services, 73–74
governance of, 55
history of, 45–46, 47–48
length of stay, 47
mission oriented, 58–59, 72
outpatient departments, 69–70
ownership of, 47
as proprietary enterprises, 14
public general, 56
role in health care system, 45
service, development of, 134
size of, 47
structure of, 52–56
Hospital Insurance Association, on national health insurance, 171
Hospital Statistics, 46
Hospital Survey and Construction Act (1946), 50, 111, 134–135, 136
''Hospitalist,'' 30, 65
House Un-American Activities Committee, 151
Human immunodeficiency virus (HIV) infection, 5
Human response, in nursing, 34–35
Hypertension, major cause of morbidity, 5

Ill-health, social factors of, 5
Illegitimacy, in Mississippi, 132
Indemnity health insurance, 148
Independent Practice Association (IPA), 147, 151, 154,
Independent Practice Organization (IPO), 156

Indian Health Service, 111, 113
Industrial health service units, 78–79
Infant mortality rate, 4–5
Infections control committee, 54
Influenza, 5
Information system specialists, health care, 26
Inhalation therapy, 55
Injuries, 5
Inpatient care, physicians, 29
Institute of Medicine, 105, 139
Institutions, health care, 6, 7, 84
Insurance companies, as proprietary enterprises, 15
Integrated Delivery System (IDS), 158–160
Internal medicine, 53, 68

Japan
- infant mortality rate, 4
- national health care system, 4–5, 167

Joint conference committee, 54
Judiciary, government role in health care, 108

Kaiser Foundation Health Plans of Northern and Southern California, 160
Kaiser-Permanente, 149
Kidney disease, leading cause of death, 5
Knowledge and personnel production, health care, 6, 8, 84
Koop, C. Everett, on managed care, 144

Labor Department, health care role, 110, 116
Laboratory, hospital division, 55
Latino, medical school admissions, 33
Legislative branch, government role in health care, 107–108
Liaison Committee on Medical Education, 32
Licensed practical nurses (LPNs), 36. *See also* Nursing services
Licensed vocational nurses (LVN), 36. *See also* Nursing services
Licensing, state role in, 118
Life expectancy, in United States, 4
Local government, as health care provider, 109, 118–119
Local health department (LHD), 118–119
Local role in health care, 75–76
Long-term care hospital, 47
Long-term care, 59–60
Luft, Harold, HMO basic characteristics, 152–153

Macro health planning, 123, 124
Magnetic resonance imaging (MRI), 53
Managed care, 155–156, 157–158
- advantages of, 145
- decline in hospital beds, 50, 51
- disadvantages of, 145–146
- emergency visits, 70
- future predictions, 161–162
- health service fundor, 88, 92
- impact on
  - health care costs, 85, 101
  - hospital-medical staff arrangement, 54
  - medical specialization, 31–32
  - nursing, 39
  - physician, 28–29, 30
  - private practice, 16
- in mid-1990s, 160
- as proprietary enterprise, 15

Managed care organization (MCO), 144–145
- forms of, 156–157
- growth of, 3
- resource allocation, 3–4

Marine Hospital Service (MHS), 111
Medicaid
- expenditures, 97–98
- health service fundor, 88
- long-term care, 60
- outpatient coverage, 70
- passage of, 171
- services provided, 97

Medical departments, of hospital, 52–53

Medical education
  nurses, 35
  physician's, 32–33
Medical employment
  nurses, 35–36, 41
  physician assistant, 41
  physicians, 27–28
Medical Practice Act, New York, 26–27
Medical records, 26, 55
Medical school, 32–33
Medical specialization, growth of, 27–28, 30–32, 65
Medical staff committees, 54
Medical technology systems, 8
"Medically indigent," 97
"Medically needy," 111
Medicare, 93
  expenditures, 96
  health service fundor, 88
  and managed care, 160
  passage of, 171
  permanent rescue of, 96
  program, 93, 96–97
  spending on, 8
Mental health centers, personnel of, 41
Mental health, public health agencies, 75
Mental illness, delivery system, 17–18
Metropolitan Life, health insurance, 92
Micro health planning, 123, 124
Microbial agents, 5
Midwifery, 26
Mississippi, 132
"Moral means test," 114
Morbidity
  causes of, 5
  measure of population health status, 130–131
Mortality
  indices, 130
  measure of population health status, 130

National Association of Manufacturers, 167, 176
National Cancer Institute, 112
National Center for Health Statistics, 51, 112, 117
National Council on Health Planning and Development, 138
National health care, systems of, 4–5
National health insurance, 165, 166–173
  1980s, 172–173
  1960s and 1970s, 171–172
  current proposals, 176
  world wide, 167
National Health Board, 179, 180
National Health Planning and Resource Development Act, 136
National Health Service Corps, 78, 111, 183
National Heart, Lung, and Blood Institutes, 112
National Hospital Discharge Survey, 51
National Institute of Occupational Safety and Health (NIOSH), 115–116
National Institutes of Health (NIH), 98, 111, 112–113
National Leadership Commission on Health, 176
Native Americans, medical school admissions, 33
Natural Resources Defense Council, 109
"Need," defined as, 130
Neighborhood Health Centers (NHCs), 65, 68, 76–78
"Neighborhood health worker," 77
Neurology, hospital department, 53
Neurosurgery, hospital department, 53
"NHI by contract," 173, 174
Nightingale, Florence, 35
Nurse extender (NE), 37
Nurse practitioner, 26, 37–38
Nurses
  employment of, 35–36, 41
  extent of, 35
  number of, 25
Nurses' aides, 36. *See also* Nursing services
Nursing, 34–39, 35, 37
Nursing homes, 9, 14, 60

Nursing Practice Act of New York State, 34–35
Nursing services, 36
education for, 35, 36
expanded role of, 37–38
in military, 35
shortage in, 38–39
Nurturing, 35
Nutrition, hospital division, 55
Nutritional standards, set by Department of Agriculture, 13
Nutritionists and dieticians, 26

Objectives, of health planning, 125, 132
Obstetrics and gynecology, 53, 68
Occupancy rate
hospital, 48, 49
nursing homes, 60
Occupational Safety and Health Administration (OSHA), 13, 15, 115–116
Occupational therapy, 55
Office of Disease Prevention and Health Promotion (ODPAP), 113, 138
Office of Economic Opportunity, 76
Oil, Chemical, and Atomic Workers, 176
Ophthalmology, 53, 68
Optometrists, 25, 26
Orthopedic impairments, 5
Orthopedics, 53, 68
Osteopathic medical schools, 32
Otolaryngology, 53
Out-of-pocket expenditures, 92–93
Outcomes, 126
Outpatient departments (OPDs), 69, 71–72. *See also* Clinic services

PacifiCare, 160
"Pain management," 53
Patient visits, 68–69, 70, 73
Pauper stigma, 105
Pediatrics, 53, 68
Pennsylvania Hospital, 46
Pepper Commission, on U.S. health care system, 20, 176
Per episode of care, payment mode, 99
Per unit of care, payment mode, 99
Personal health care, 98
Personal Health Care System, 173–175
Personnel
in health care field, 25–26
in primary care, 66–67
physicians in teaching hospitals, 71–72
Personnel, health care, 6, 7, 84
national expenditures for, 98–99
"Pesthouse," 46
Pharmaceutical use, physicians role in, 3
Pharmacists, 25, 41–42
Pharmacy, 55
Pharmacy and therapeutics committee, 54–55
Physical therapists, 25, 26
Physical therapy, 55
Physician(s), 25
changing position of, 7
employment of, 27–28
impact on hospital, 54
licensure, 26–27
over-supply of, 31
population ratio, 28
primary care, 66–67
Physician Assistant (PA), 39–41
education of, 40–41
employment of, 41
licensure of, 40
role of, 40
Physician-hospital organization (PHO), 54
Physicians for a National Health Program, 176
Podiatrists, 25, 26
Point-of-Service arrangement, 93, 155, 157
Portable coverage, 180
Precertification, 156
Preferred provider organization (PPO), 156, 180
Prenatal care, public health agencies, 75
Prepaid group practice (PPGP), 77, 148–151
advantages of, 150–151

Prepaid group practice *(continued)*
forms of, 149–150
Primary care, 16, 63–67. *See also* Ambulatory care
and health delivery system, 67
history of, 65–66
personnel for, 66–67
public health agencies, 76
Prison, health services, 68
Private entrepreneurial model, 3. *See also* Private practice
Private insurance, health service fundor, 88
Private practice, 15–16, 28–29
Program evaluation technique, 11
Program planning, 132–133
Proprietary health services enterprises, 14–15
Psychiatric hospitals, 47, 48t
Psychiatry, 53
Psychologists, 41
Public health
agency services, 75–76
centers, personnel of, 41
current problems in, 119
services, 108
Public-general hospital, 56
Public Health Service (PHS), 110, 111–113
Public Health Service Act Amendments (1966), 136
Public Law 89–239, volunteerism, 136

Radiology, 53
Radiotherapy, 53, 55
Rationing, 177
Red label, PPGP, 151
Reform package of 1985, 173
Regional medical complexes, 135
Regional Medical Program (RMP), 135, 136, 159
"Regionalization," 134
Registered care technician (RCT), 36
Registered nurse population ratio, 35
Registered nurses (RNs), 36. *See also* Nursing services
Rehabilitation therapy, hospital division, 55
"Roemer's Law," 51
Rosenfeld, Leonard, on health planning approaches, 124, 128

Satellite OPD, 74
School health centers, personnel of, 41, 68
School health clinics, 79–80
Secondary care, 17
Sedentary lifestyle, 5
Sexual behavior, 5
Sexually transmitted diseases (STDs), 75
Short term care hospital, 47, 48
Sickness Insurance Act, 166
"Social/community market," 2–3
Social Security Act, Medicaid, 93, 97–98
Social Security Act (1935), passage of, 104, 169
Social Security Administration, 110
Social services, 55
Social workers, 25, 41
Speech therapy, 55
"Spend down," 97
Staff model, 149, 154
State government, as health care provider, 109, 116–118
State health agency (SHAs) programs, 117
State Health Planning and Development Agencies, 138
State health programs, 117
Stroke, 5, 135
Substance Abuse and Mental Health Service Administration (SAMHSA), 111, 113
Suicide, 5
Supplementary Security Income (SSI), 97
Surgeon General, 111
Surgery, major hospital medical department, 53
Surgical group, in clinics, 71
Surgi-centers, 74

Surgical interventions, physicians role in, 3
Switzerland, national health care system, 4–5

Taft, Robert, Sr., 169–170, 171
Tenth Amendment, U. S. Constitution, 106–108
Terborg, James, on worksite health promotion, 79
Tertiary care, 17
"Third-party payor," 9, 28, 71, 88
Tissue committee, 55
Title XVIII, of Social Security Act, 93
Title XIX, of Social Security Act, 97
Tobacco regulation, 112
Tobacco use, 5
Toxic agents, 5
Trauma system, need for, 75
Travelers, health insurance, 92
Treating, in nursing, 34
Tuberculosis (TB), 18, 76
"Tyranny of the bed," 58

United States
- health care services, spending on, 1, 8–9
- history of health care role, 103–106
- population of, 4
- role in health care, 103–106
- socioeconomic problems in the, 4

United States Constitution, 106
United States, health care system, 1–2, 6, 65
- current state of, 21–22, 100–101
- future of, 181–183
- government role in, 12–13
- market system, 2, 3
- organization of, 10–16

United States Preventive Services Task Force, 113
Unmet needs, 131–132
Upper respiratory infections, 5
Urology, 53
Utilization review, 161

"Value free planning," 128
Values, and health planning, 128–129
Veterans Affairs, Department of, 12
- health care role, 110, 114–115
- health program, 98

Visiting Nurse Association, 14
Voluntary agencies, 13–14
- funding of, 88
- role of, 109

"War on poverty," 76
Welfare Repeal Act of 1996, 97
White Americans
- home health care, 80
- infant mortality rate, 5
- life expectancy, 4
- patient visits, 68, 70, 73

Women
- medical school admissions, 33
- patient visits, 68, 70

Women and Infants Care (WIC), 115
Work-site health promotion, 78

X-ray, 53